T0383333

Pediatric Ophthalmology

Editor

MARY LOU MCGREGOR

PEDIATRIC CLINICS
OF NORTH AMERICA

www.pediatric.theclinics.com

Consulting Editor
BONITA F. STANTON

June 2014 • Volume 61 • Number 3

ELSEVIER

1600 John F. Kennedy Boulevard • Suite 1800 • Philadelphia, Pennsylvania, 19103-2899

http://www.theclinics.com

THE PEDIATRIC CLINICS OF NORTH AMERICA Volume 61, Number 3
June 2014 ISSN 0031-3955, ISBN-13: 978-0-323-29928-2

Editor: Kerry Holland
Developmental Editor: Casey Jackson

The Pediatric Clinics of North America (ISSN 0031-3955) is published bimonthly by Elsevier Inc., 360 Park Avenue South, New York, NY 10010-1710. Months of issue are February, April, June, August, October, and December. Periodicals postage paid at New York, NY and additional mailing offices. Subscription prices are $200.00 per year (US individuals), $493.00 per year (US institutions), $270.00 per year (Canadian individuals), $657.00 per year (Canadian institutions), $325.00 per year (international individuals), $657.00 per year (international institutions), $100.00 per year (US students and residents), and $165.00 per year (international and Canadian residents and students). To receive students/resident rare, orders must be accompanied by name of affiliated institution, date of term, and the signature of program/residency coordinator on institution letterhead. Orders will be billed at individual rate until proof of status is received. Foreign air speed delivery is included in all Clinics subscription prices. All prices are subject to change without notice. **POSTMASTER:** Send address changes to The Pediatric Clinics of North America, Elsevier Health Sciences Division, Subscription Customer Service, 3251 Riverport Lane, Maryland Heights, MO 63043. **Customer Service: 1-800-654-2452 (US and Canada). From outside of the US and Canada: 1-314-447-8871. Fax: 1-314-447-8029. For print support, E-mail: JournalsCustomerService-usa@elsevier.com. For online support, E-mail: JournalsOnlineSupport-usa@elsevier.com.**

Reprints. For copies of 100 or more, of articles in this publication, please contact the Commercial Reprints Department, Elsevier Inc., 360 Park Avenue South, New York, NY 10010-1710. Tel.: 212-633-3874; Fax: 212-633-3820; E-mail: reprints@elsevier.com.

The Pediatric Clinics of North America is also published in Spanish by McGraw-Hill Inter-americana Editores S.A., Mexico City, Mexico; in Portuguese by Riechmann and Affonso Editores, Rua Comandante Coelho 1085, CEP 21250, Rio de Janeiro, Brazil; and in Greek by Althayia SA, Athens, Greece.

The Pediatric Clinics of North America is covered in MEDLINE/PubMed (Index Medicus), Excerpta Medica, Current Contents, Current Contents/Clinical Medicine, Science Citation Index, ASCA, ISI/BIOMED, and BIOSIS.

PROGRAM OBJECTIVE

The goal of the *Pediatric Clinics of North America* is to keep practicing physicians and residents up to date with current clinical practice in pediatrics by providing timely articles reviewing the state-of-the-art in patient care.

TARGET AUDIENCE

All practicing pediatricians, physicians and healthcare professionals who provide patient care to pediatric patients.

LEARNING OBJECTIVES

Upon completion of this activity, participants will be able to:
1. Review pediatric idiopathic intracranial hypertension.
2. Discuss ocular diseases and disorders including allergic eye disease, pediatric red eye, amblyopia, genetic disorders, periocular hemangiomas and lymphangiomas, as well as retinopathy of prematurity.
3. Explain various ocular therapies including pediatric refractive surgery and vision therapy for convergence insufficiency.

ACCREDITATION

The Elsevier Office of Continuing Medical Education (EOCME) is accredited by the Accreditation Council for Continuing Medical Education (ACCME) to provide continuing medical education for physicians.

The EOCME designates this enduring material for a maximum of 15 *AMA PRA Category 1 Credit*(s)™. Physicians should claim only the credit commensurate with the extent of their participation in the activity.

All other health care professionals requesting continuing education credit for this enduring material will be issued a certificate of participation.

DISCLOSURE OF CONFLICTS OF INTEREST

The EOCME assesses conflict of interest with its instructors, faculty, planners, and other individuals who are in a position to control the content of CME activities. All relevant conflicts of interest that are identified are thoroughly vetted by EOCME for fair balance, scientific objectivity, and patient care recommendations. EOCME is committed to providing its learners with CME activities that promote improvements or quality in healthcare and not a specific proprietary business or a commercial interest.

The planning committee, staff, authors and editors listed below have identified no financial relationships or relationships to products or devices they or their spouse/life partner have with commercial interest related to the content of this CME activity:

William Anninger, MD; Charline S. Boente, MD, MS; Diana DeSantis, BA, MD; Richard P. Golden, MD; Kerry Holland; Brynne Hunter; Catherine O. Jordan, MD; Aaron R. Kaufman, BA; Indu Kumari; Mary Lou McGregor, MD; Jill McNair; Virginia Miraldi Utz, MD; Ken K. Nischal, MD, FRCOphth; Christina N. Nye, MD; Faruk H. Örge, MD; Lindsay Parnell; Rachel E. Reem, MD; David L. Rogers, MD; Hannah L. Scanga, MD, CGC; Erin D. Stahl, MD; Bonita F. Stanton, MD; Melissa M. Wong, MD.

The planning committee, staff, authors and editors listed below have identified financial relationships or relationships to products or devices they or their spouse/life partner have with commercial interest related to the content of this CME activity:

UNAPPROVED/OFF-LABEL USE DISCLOSURE

The EOCME requires CME faculty to disclose to the participants:
1. When products or procedures being discussed are off-label, unlabelled, experimental, and/or investigational (not US Food and Drug Administration (FDA) approved); and
2. Any limitations on the information presented, such as data that are preliminary or that represent ongoing research, interim analyses, and/or unsupported opinions. Faculty may discuss information about pharmaceutical agents that is outside of FDA-approved labelling. This information is intended solely for CME and is not intended to promote off-label use of these medications. If you have any questions, contact the medical affairs department of the manufacturer for the most recent prescribing information.

TO ENROLL

To enroll in the *Pediatric Clinics of North America* Continuing Medical Education program, call customer service at 1-800-654-2452 or sign up online at http://www.theclinics.com/home/cme. The CME program is available to subscribers for an additional annual fee of USD 261.

METHOD OF PARTICIPATION

In order to claim credit, participants must complete the following:

1. Complete enrolment as indicated above.
2. Read the activity.
3. Complete the CME Test and Evaluation. Participants must achieve a score of 70% on the test. All CME Tests and Evaluations must be completed online.

CME INQUIRIES/SPECIAL NEEDS

For all CME inquiries or special needs, please contact elsevierCME@elsevier.com.

Contributors

CONSULTING EDITOR

BONITA F. STANTON, MD
Vice Dean for Research and Professor of Pediatrics, School of Medicine, Wayne State University, Detroit, Michigan

EDITOR

MARY LOU MCGREGOR, MD
Associate Clinical Professor of Ophthalmology, Ohio State University; Director, Ophthalmology Clinic, Nationwide Children's Hospital, Columbus, Ohio

AUTHORS

WILLIAM ANNINGER, MD
Department of Ophthalmology, The Children's Hospital of Philadelphia, Philadelphia, Pennsylvania

CHARLINE S. BOENTE, MD, MS
Department of Ophthalmology and Visual Sciences, University Hospitals Rainbow Babies and Children's Hospital, Case Western Reserve University, Cleveland, Ohio

DIANA DESANTIS, MD
Children's Eye Physicians, Denver, Colorado

RICHARD P. GOLDEN, MD
Clinical Assistant Professor, Department of Ophthalmology, Nationwide Children's Hospital and The Ohio State University, Columbus, Ohio

CATHERINE O. JORDAN, MD
Department of Ophthalmology, Nationwide Children's Hospital, Columbus, Ohio

AARON R. KAUFMAN, BA
Boston University School of Medicine, Boston, Massachusetts

MARY LOU MCGREGOR, MD
Associate Clinical Professor of Ophthalmology, Ohio State University; Director, Ophthalmology Clinic, Nationwide Children's Hospital, Columbus, Ohio

VIRGINIA MIRALDI UTZ, MD, FAAP
Assistant Professor Educator-Affiliate, Department of Ophthalmology, University of Cinncinati; Assistant Professor of Ophthalmology, Abrahamson Eye Institute, Cincinnati Children's Hospital Medical Center, Cincinnati, Ohio

KEN K. NISCHAL, MD, FRCOphth
UPMC Eye Center, University of Pittsburgh; Children's Eye Center, Children's Hospital of Pittsburgh of UPMC, Pittsburgh, Pennsylvania

CHRISTINA NYE, MD
Northwest Pediatric Ophthalmology, Spokane, Washington

FARUK H. ÖRGE, MD
Department of Ophthalmology and Visual Sciences, University Hospitals Rainbow Babies and Children's Hospital, Case Western Reserve University, Cleveland, Ohio

RACHEL E. REEM, MD
Pediatric Ophthalmology Fellow, Department of Ophthalmology, Nationwide Children's Hospital, Columbus, Ohio

DAVID L. ROGERS, MD
Department of Ophthalmology, Nationwide Children's Hospital, The Ohio State University College of Medicine, Columbus, Ohio

HANNAH L. SCANGA, MS, CGC
UPMC Eye Center, University of Pittsburgh; Children's Eye Center, Children's Hospital of Pittsburgh of UPMC, Pittsburgh, Pennsylvania

ERIN D. STAHL, MD
Pediatric Ophthalmologist, Children's Mercy Hospitals and Clinics; Assistant Professor of Pediatric Ophthalmology, University of Missouri-Kansas City, Kansas City, Missouri; Assistant Clinical Professor, Department of Ophthalmology, University of Kansas, Prairie Village, Kansas

MELISSA M. WONG, MD
Department of Ophthalmology, The Children's Hospital of Philadelphia, Philadelphia, Pennsylvania

Contents

> Implementing standard vision screening techniques in the primary care practice is the most effective means to detect children with potential vision problems at an age when the vision loss may be treatable. A critical period of vision development occurs in the first few weeks of life; thus, it is imperative that serious problems are detected at this time. Although it is not possible to quantitate an infant's vision, evaluating ocular health appropriately can mean the difference between sight and blindness and, in the case of retinoblastoma, life or death.

> Amblyopia refers to unilateral or bilateral reduction in best corrected visual acuity, not directly attributed to structural abnormality of the eye or posterior visual pathways. Early detection of amblyopia is crucial to obtaining the best response to treatment. Amblyopia responds best to treatment in the first few years of life. In the past several years a series of studies undertaken by the Pediatric Eye Disease Investigator Group (PEDIG) have been designed to evaluate traditional methods for treating amblyopia and provide evidence on which to base treatment decisions. This article summarizes and discusses the findings of the PEDIG studies to date.

> This article reviews current thoughts regarding pediatric refractive surgery. This encompasses current trends in adult refractive surgery, differences between adult and pediatric refractive surgery, and future possibilities for refractive technology for the pediatric population.

> The lacrimal system comprises of a series of anatomical structures with specific physiologic properties. Tearing from a nasolacrimal duct obstruction (NLDO) is the most common lacrimal system abnormality encountered by pediatric ophthalmologists. Most NLDOs spontaneously improve with

pediatric patients have largely been based on the adult literature. Exciting new evidence is now available to assist the clinician in managing pediatric patients with IIH.

PEDIATRIC CLINICS OF NORTH AMERICA

Foreword

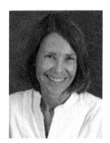

Bonita F. Stanton, MD
Consulting Editor

All five of the "traditional" senses—sight, hearing, smell, taste, touch—are critical to a child's development and to functioning, as a child and an adult. Globally, in both 1990 and 2010, using the current WHO definition, approximately 32 million persons worldwide were blind.[1] Although adults over the age of fifty years represented nearly two-thirds of those with visual impairment,[2] an estimated 1.4 million children globally were blind.[3]

Of course, any decrease in visual acuity can impact development and functioning. The global burden of visual difficulties is not evenly distributed; there is overwhelming evidence that rates are inversely related to national socioeconomic status.[3,4] Within the United States, there is also evidence of higher rates of visual impairment among groups with fewer resources. Therefore, both within the United States and across the globe, pediatricians must be aware of conditions and circumstances that can threaten vision, available preventive measures, and new therapies for treatment.

As the authors describe in this outstanding volume dedicated to vision in children, great strides have been made in recent years in preventing and identifying any loss of visual acuity, and, when identified, correcting it. The articles are written for the practicing pediatrician and thus describe conditions that you may detect in your practice and/or about which parents and patients may be knowledgeable and have questions.

Bonita F. Stanton, MD
School of Medicine
Wayne State University
1261 Scott Hall
540 East Canfield, Suite 1261
Detroit, MI 48201, USA

E-mail address:
bstanton@med.wayne.edu

http://dx.doi.org/10.1016/j.pcl.2014.03.013
0031-3955/14/$ – see front matter © 2014 Published by Elsevier Inc.
pediatric.theclinics.com

REFERENCES

1. Stevens GA, White RA, Flaxman SR, et al, Vision Loss Expert Group. Global prevalence of vision impairment and blindness: magnitude and temporal trends, 1990-2010. Ophthalmology 2013;120(12):2377–84.
2. Pascolini D, Mariotti SP. Global estimates of visual impairment: 2010. Br J Ophthalmol 2012;96(5):614–8.
3. Courtright P, Hutchinson AK, Lewallen S. Visual impairment in children in middle- and lower-income countries. Arch Dis Child 2011;96(12):1129–34.
4. Freeman EE, Roy-Gagnon MH, Samson E, et al. The global burden of visual difficulty in low, middle, and high income countries. PLoS One 2013;8(5):e63315.

Preface

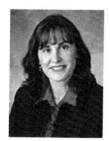

Mary Lou McGregor, MD
Editor

I relied on many wonderful colleagues to contribute to this edition of *Pediatric Clinics of North America.* I would like to acknowledge all of them for their expertise and dedication to the field of pediatric ophthalmology. Although the theme of this issue is, "What Is New in Pediatric Ophthalmology," the theme of the collection of authors was "Reconnecting with Friends and Colleagues." I am sincerely indebted to all of them.

Dr Leonard Nelson was the guest editor of the "Pediatric Ophthalmology" issue of *Pediatric Clinics of North America* in 1993. He emphasized the "importance of careful clinical evaluation" as the foundation for treating pediatric ophthalmologic disorders. The same is true twenty years later. Other fields of ophthalmology can often rely on new advanced technology to make a diagnosis, but it will always be a challenge to get a two- or a five-year-old child to cooperate with an exam or a test; therefore, the pediatrician and ophthalmologist must often rely on their clinical skills. The ophthalmologist and pediatrician must continue to work as a team in taking care of children with eye disease.

I would like to thank Casey Jackson and Kerry Holland, editors at Elsevier; Dr Bonita Stanton, consulting editor; along with all of the publishing staff at Elsevier for their patience and help. They are amazing at what they do, and I am grateful to have had the opportunity to work with them. I want to thank my family for their patience and much needed technological help. I would like to acknowledge Drs Hiram Hardesty, William Annable, Gary Rogers, Don Bremer, and John Lee. These ophthalmologists were patient enough to train me in the field of pediatric ophthalmology and strabismus, but more importantly, they inspired me to want to teach.

Mary Lou McGregor, MD
Ophthalmology Clinic
Nationwide Children's Hospital
OCC Suite 4C
700 Children's Drive
Columbus, OH 43205, USA

E-mail address:
mlkmcgregor@gmail.com

A Child's Vision

KEYWORDS

- Red reflex • Nystagmus • Cortical vision impairment • Delayed visual maturation
- Vision screening • Instrument-based screeners

KEY POINTS

- Implementing standard vision screening techniques in the primary care practice is the most effective means to detect children with potential vision problems at an age when the vision loss may be treatable.
- A critical period of vision development occurs in the first few weeks of life; thus, it is imperative that serious problems are detected at this time.
- Although it is not possible to quantitate an infant's vision, evaluating ocular health appropriately can mean the difference between sight and blindness and, in the case of retinoblastoma, life or death.

INTRODUCTION

In the United States, an estimated 1 in 20 children is at risk for permanent vision loss.[1,2] Amblyopia is the most common cause of vision loss. Other causes of vision loss include cortical vision impairment, delayed visual maturation, nystagmus, Retinopathy of prematurity, cataracts, glaucoma, optic nerve hypoplasia, and retinal abnormalities. All of these conditions can be discovered with appropriate knowledge regarding assessing visual behavior in children. The most important aspect of discovering vision abnormalities is understanding and assessing a child's visual behavior by the primary care provider at every well-child visit. In theory, this approach is the most effective screening for the largest number of children because most children see their primary care provider several times during infancy and early childhood.

Because a critical period of vision development occurs in the first few weeks of life, it is imperative that serious problems are detected at this time. Although it is not possible to quantitate an infant's vision, evaluating ocular health appropriately can mean the difference between sight and blindness and, in the case of retinoblastoma, life or death.

WHAT IS NORMAL VISUAL BEHAVIOR?

The first few weeks of life are a critical time for vision development. During this critical period, visual acuity develops rapidly and depends on a visual stimulus that is equal

---

Northwest Pediatric Ophthalmology, 105 West 8th Avenue, Suite 512, Spokane, WA 99204, USA
E-mail address: nwpo.nye@gmail.com

Pediatr Clin N Am 61 (2014) 495–503
http://dx.doi.org/10.1016/j.pcl.2014.03.001
0031-3955/14/$ – see front matter © 2014 Elsevier Inc. All rights reserved.

pediatric.theclinics.com

and focused in each eye.[3-5] A full-term infant should be adverse to bright light when introduced to each eye separately. The infant should consistently blink to light with each eye individually. Evaluating the normal infantile reflex of opening the eyes when the lights are turned off and closing when turned on is very important to note. Convergence spasms, or intermittent esotropia, are common in infants. This intermittent esotropia usually resolve completely by 3 to 4 months of age but occasionally lasts until 6 months.

Infants are typically able to fix on objects by 4 to 6 weeks of age. By 2 to 3 months of age, an infant should be able to follow objects.[6,7] By 3 years of age, most children can identify character shapes using Allen figures or Lea symbols, with each eye checked separately.[8] A child should be able to see 20/40 by 4 years of age and 20/30 by 5 years of age with each eye. By 5 years of age, most children can identify Snellen letters. Although, the classic end point for vision development is about 9 years of age, new multicenter controlled clinical research study has extended this period to as late as 13 to 17 years of age.[9] Normative visual acuity data for children aged 3 to 10 years have recently been published (**Table 1**).[10,11]

HOW TO ASSESS AN INFANT'S VISION

When evaluating an infant, look at eyelid structure and contour, conjunctiva, irises, pupils, and red reflex. Specifically look for any eyelid colobomas or defects, dermoids or dermolipomas, iris colobomas, or pupil irregularities. Although the pupil in an infant is miotic until about a month of age, a red reflex must be elicited during the first few weeks of life. If unable to detect a red reflex, immediate referral to a pediatric ophthalmologist is essential (**Fig. 1**).

Between 4 months and 3 years of age, the best way to assess a child's vision is by observing fixation and following. Cover each eye separately and present an interesting silent object. Observe to see that the child follows the object equally and steadily with each eye. Determine if the child consistently objects to covering either eye. Always assess and compare the red reflex of each eye simultaneously. Evaluate the corneal light reflex to detect strabismus (**Fig. 2**).

An important observation is whether the child has an abnormal head posture. Pay particular attention to a child who has a consistent head turn or tilt, which may indicate strabismus or nystagmus. Evaluate the eye alignment in all gazes. The misalignment or nystagmus often becomes apparent when the child's head is placed in a different position. Refer any child with an abnormal head posture for evaluation of strabismus or nystagmus (**Fig. 3**).

By 3 to 4 years of age, it is important to test vision using a standard eye chart with pictures or letters. The child should be able to identify at least the 20/40 line with each

Table 1 Expected visual milestones through early childhood	
Age	**Visual Milestone**
Birth to 2 mo	Blinks to light
2–3 mo	Fix and follows
3 mo to 3 y	Central steady maintained
4–5 y	20/40 Pictures
5–6 y	20/30 Letters
6–7 y+	20/20 Snellen

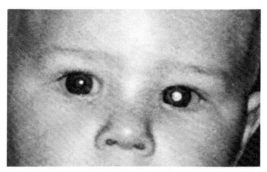

Fig. 1. A child with retinoblastoma presenting with leukocoria.

eye checked separately. It is extremely important to watch for peeking around an occluder. If a child consistently tries to peek when one eye is covered, suspect poor vision in the eye that is being tested. Equally important is to be aware of a difference between the two eyes. For instance, if a child can see 20/20 with one eye but only 20/40 with the other, refer the child for evaluation. Always assess and compare the red reflex and the corneal light reflex. Refer any child who does not meet normal criteria.

An excellent comprehensive review with suggestions and techniques on how to assess an infant or child's eyes and vision was recently published.[12]

THE RED REFLEX TEST

By far, the most effective test for detecting early abnormalities in infants and children is the Bruckner red reflex test.[13] This test is essential in evaluating the ocular health of infants and young children. The red reflex detects the light reflected back from the retina. The test should be performed with the examination lights off. Turning the lights off elicits the infantile reflex of opening the eyes and gives the examiner the largest

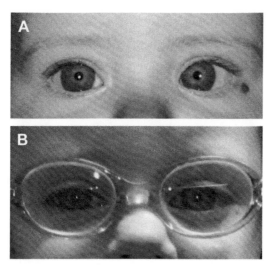

Fig. 2. (*A*) Abnormal corneal light reflex. Note the left esotropia caused by overaccommodation. (*B*) The corneal light reflex is normal when the child looks through her bifocal.

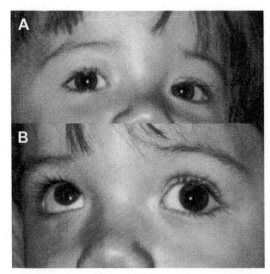

Fig. 3. (*A*) A child with a left face turn. (*B*) The strabismus is not evident until the child looks to the left.

pupil possible. The examination is performed using a direct ophthalmoscope, set at +2.00 diopters, at arm's length in the darkened room. Assess the contour of the pupil at the same time. Look for each red reflex separately and then compare both at the same time. The color of the red reflex can vary significantly from individual to individual. A lightly pigmented person will have a bright orange-red reflex, whereas a darkly pigmented person may have a red-gray reflex (**Figs. 4** and **5**).

Although an infant's pupils are miotic and the red reflex can be difficult to assess, it remains the single most important screening tool. Discovering an abnormal red reflex in the critical period of vision development is essential. Comments such as "infant is

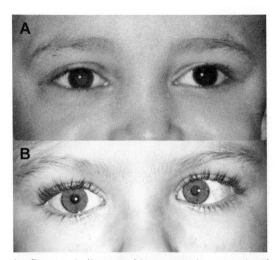

Fig. 4. Unequal red reflex may indicate strabismus or anisometropia. The color of the red reflex varies with individual's pigmentation. (*A*) Slight right esotropia. (*B*) A left esotropia. Note the brighter reflex in the deviating eye.

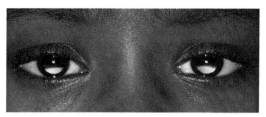

Fig. 5. A bright crescent in part of the red reflex may indicate refractive error. This child is highly myopic. Also note the color of the red reflex caused by dark pigmentation.

uncooperative," "eyelids are closed tightly," or "unable to evaluate red reflex" are absolutely unacceptable and may result in permanent vision loss or even death because of delayed treatment. Never feel content with an infant's eye examination until you are certain that a red reflex is present in each eye.

The red reflex may reveal an iris coloboma or other iris abnormality that requires referral to an ophthalmologist. A white reflex may indicate a cataract, chorioretinal coloboma, optic nerve anomaly, or a retinoblastoma. These conditions require urgent referral to an ophthalmologist. A delay in referring an infant with an abnormal red reflex often results in irreversible vision loss, loss of the eye, or even death.

In older children, comparison of the red reflex test can be used to detect refractive errors, strabismus, or media opacities. The red reflex should be equal in each eye when viewed simultaneously. If there is a difference in the red reflex, referral to an ophthalmologist is indicated.

NYSTAGMUS

Nystagmus is involuntary, conjugate, horizontal or vertical oscillating movement of the eyes.[14] It is often the first sign of visual abnormality in infants. Congenital nystagmus is a misnomer in that it typically presents between 8 and 12 weeks of age. Nystagmus should be differentiated from roving eye movements, which usually indicate significant visual impairment. Any child with nystagmus or roving eye movements should be referred to an ophthalmologist for further evaluation.

Nystagmus in an infant is typically the result of an abnormality of the anterior visual pathway as opposed to cortical or cerebral abnormality. The presence or absence of nystagmus is very important in aiding in the diagnosis of an apparently blind infant.

DELAYED VISUAL MATURATION

An important entity to consider in an infant who does not seem to see is delayed visual maturation. This term refers to an infant who does not meet visual milestones and may act essentially blind. On careful questioning, there is no significant past medical or birth history to consider cortical vision impairment. The eye examination, including refraction, retina evaluation, and optic nerves, is entirely normal. Usually by 6 to 9 months of age, the child will spontaneously begin to see and will rapidly develop normal visual behavior. The diagnosis can only be suspected early on and confirmed in retrospect once the child begins to behave visually normally.[15]

CORTICAL VISION IMPAIRMENT

An infant who is not fixing and following objects by 3 to 4 months of age requires evaluation. Occasionally, some of these children suffer from visual maturation delay as discussed, and within a few more months the vision seems to be normal. If normal development does not occur, more investigation is needed. As discussed, if nystagmus or roving eye movements are present, an abnormality in the anterior vision pathway is suspected. If there is a lack of nystagmus, the abnormality likely lies in the posterior pathways or visual cortex. Although once referred to as cortical blindness, most clinicians and researchers now prefer the term *cortical vision impairment* or *cerebral vision impairment*. Most infants and children affected by CVI show a degree of residual vision and are not totally blind.[16,17]

There are several common causes of CVI. The most common is hypoxic/ischemic brain injury.[18] Ischemic brain damage may occur any time in the perinatal period or after birth, following cardiac or respiratory arrest. Periventricular or intraventricular hemorrhages are particularly common in premature infants. Head trauma, meningitis, cerebral malformations, and hydrocephalus are other causes of ischemic injury in infants and young children.

An infant with cortical vision impairment may act essentially blind and will not meet the normal visual milestones. Examination of the eyes typically reveals no abnormalities. The pupils usually respond to light, and there is no nystagmus. The infant simply does not respond normally to visually stimuli. During early childhood, there is often improvement in overall visual function; but the rate of improvement is slower than normal.[19]

VISION SCREENING

The American Association for Pediatric Ophthalmology and Strabismus has developed recommended screening guidelines based on a child's age. In addition, the American Academy of Pediatrics, the American Association of Certified Orthoptists, the American Academy of Ophthalmology, and the American Association of Pediatric Ophthalmology and Strabismus jointly recommend age-appropriate vision screening by the primary care provider for all children before discharge from the nursery, at 6 months of age, at 3 to 4 years of age, and annually for school-aged children (**Table 2**).[20]

There are several important reasons to include vision screenings in the child's medical home during well-child visits. First of all, this is the best opportunity to potentially screen the entire pediatric population. Secondly, a medically trained professional has the knowledge to assess visual behavior in the context of overall development. Thirdly, it provides an effective setting for early and frequent screenings. Additionally, it is cost-effective for the parent, both in time and money. An understanding of the seriousness of potential medical problems is essential in the timely and appropriate referral to a pediatric ophthalmologist.

There are efforts in some states to enforce mandatory eye examinations. Although this may seem like a good idea, this is not supported by the American Academy of Ophthalmology or the American Association of Pediatric Ophthalmology and Strabismus for several reasons. First of all, the examiner may have little to no medical training. Secondly, a solitary eye examination may not be sufficient to detect childhood eye problems. A single eye examination would provide a false sense of security that all is well. Additionally, there are valid concerns that a mandatory eye examination would result in overprescribing of spectacles.[21]

As of this writing, most but not all states require vision screening of school-aged children. Requirements vary from state to state.[22]

INSTRUMENTS FOR VISION SCREENING

An important advancement of vision screening is the development of instruments for objective vision assessment in the preverbal child. A recent study found that the use of

Table 2
Vision screening recommendations

Age	Tests	Referral Criteria Comments
Newborn to 6 mo	Ocular history Vision assessment External inspection of the eyes and lids Ocular motility assessment Pupil examination Red reflex examination	Refer infants who do not track well after 3 mo of age. Refer infants with an abnormal red reflex or history of retinoblastoma in a parent or sibling.
6 to 42 mo	Ocular history Vision assessment External inspection of the eyes and lids Ocular motility assessment Pupil examination Red reflex examination Visual acuity testing Objective screening device photoscreening Ophthalmoscopy	Refer infants with strabismus. Refer infants with chronic tearing or discharge. Refer children who fail photoscreening.
42 mo to 5 y	Ocular history Vision assessment External inspection of the eyes and lids Ocular motility assessment Pupil examination Red reflex examination Visual acuity testing (preferred) or photoscreening Ophthalmoscopy	Refer children who cannot read at least 20/40 with either eye. They must be able to identify most of the optotypes on the 20/40 line. Refer children who fail photoscreening.
5 y and older[a]	Ocular history Vision assessment External inspection of the eyes and lids Ocular motility assessment Pupil examination Red reflex examination Visual acuity testing Ophthalmoscopy	Refer children who cannot read at least 20/32 with either eye. They must be able to identify most of the optotypes on the 20/32 line. Refer children who are not reading at grade level.

[a] Repeat screening every 1 to 2 years after 5 years of age.

instruments in vision screening in infants and toddlers resulted in earlier detection of amblyopia.[23,24] Essential characteristics of an instrument for screening are accuracy, reproducibility, ease of use, and fast acting. The most common instruments on the market today are photoscreeners and autorefractors. A photoscreener images the red reflex to detect refractive errors, media opacities, and strabismus. Autorefractors detect refractive errors only and do not evaluate media opacities or strabismus. The technology of these devices is progressing rapidly. In the upcoming years, there will likely be affordable, easy-to-use, and accurate hand-held devices, which can be implemented as part of the screening process in the primary care physician's office. It is imperative that these instruments be used in conjunction with, and not in lieu of, a skilled medical eye screening by the primary care provider.

SUMMARY

In conclusion, implementing standard vision screening techniques in the primary care practice is the most effective means to detect children with potential vision problems at an age when the vision loss may be treatable.

REFERENCES

1. Friedman DS, Repka M, Katz J, et al. Prevalence of amblyopia and strabismus in white and African American children aged 6 through 71 months, the Baltimore Pediatric Eye Disease Study. Ophthalmology 2009;116(11): 2128–34.
2. Why save sight? Children's Eye Foundation Web site. Copyright 2013. Available at: www.childrenseyefoundation.org/index.php/why-save-sight/why-save-sight. Accessed January 30, 2014.
3. Hainline L, Riddell P, Grose-Fifer J, et al. Development of accommodation and convergence in infancy. Behav Brain Res 1992;49:33–50.
4. Taylor D, Avetisov S. Normal and abnormal visual development. In: Pediatric ophthalmology. Boston: Blackwell Scientific Publications; 1990. p. 12–5.
5. Wright KW. Pediatric eye examination. Pediatric ophthalmology and strabismus. St Louis (MO): Mosby; 1995. p. 57–62.
6. Currie DC, Manny RE. The development of accommodation. Vision Res 1997; 37(11):1525–33.
7. Weinacht S, Kind C, Monting J, et al. Visual development in preterm and full-term infants: a prospective masked study. Invest Ophthalmol Vis Sci 1999;40(2): 346–53.
8. Graf MH, Becker R, Kaufmann H. Lea symbols: visual acuity assessment and detection of amblyopia. Graefes Arch Clin Exp Ophthalmol 2000;238:53.
9. Scheiman MM, Hertle RW, Beck RW. Randomized trial of treatment of amblyopia in children aged 7 to 17 years. Arch Ophthalmol 2005;123:437–47.
10. Drover JR, Felius J, Cheng CS, et al. Normative pediatric visual acuity using single surrounded HOTV optotypes on the Electronic Visual Acuity Tester following the Amblyopia Treatment Study Protocol. J AAPOS 2008;12(2):145–9.
11. Hargadon DD, Wood J, Twelker JD, et al. Recognition acuity, grating acuity, contrast sensitivity, and visual fields in 6-year-old children. Arch Ophthalmol 2010;128(1):70–4.
12. Prentiss KA, Dorfman DH. Pediatric ophthalmology in the emergency department. Emerg Med Clin North Am 2008;26:181–98.
13. Tongue A, Cibis G. Bruckner test. Am J Ophthalmol 1981;88:1041–4.
14. Brodsky MC, Baker RS, Hamed LM. Nystagmus in infancy and childhood. In: Brodsky MC, Baker RS, Hamed LM, editors. Pediatric neuro-ophthalmology. New York: Springer; 1996. p. 302–47.
15. Hall D. Delayed visual maturation. Dev Med Child Neurol 1991;33(2):181.
16. Jan JE. Behavior characteristics of children with permanent cortical visual impairment. Dev Med Child Neurol 1987;29:571–6.
17. Whiting S, Jan JE, Wong PK. Permanent cortical visual impairment in children. Dev Med Child Neurol 1985;27:730–9.
18. Brodsky MC, Baker RS, Hamed LM. The apparently blind infant. In: Brodsky MC, Baker RS, Hamed LM, editors. Pediatric neuro-ophthalmology. New York: Springer; 1996. p. 11–28.
19. Lim M. Development of visual acuity in children with cerebral visual impairment. Arch Ophthalmol 2005;123(9):1215–20.

20. Committee on Practice and Ambulatory Medicine, Section on Ophthalmology. American Association of Certified Orthoptists, American Association for Pediatric Ophthalmology and Strabismus, American Academy of Ophthalmology. Eye examination in infants, children, and young adults by pediatricians. Pediatrics 2003; 111(4):902–7.
21. Donahue SP. How often are spectacles prescribed to "normal" preschool children? J AAPOS 2004;8(3):224–9.
22. State-by-state vision screening requirements. AAPOS Web site. Copyright 2014. Available at: www.aapos.org/resources/state_by_state_vision_requirements/. Accessed January 30, 2014.
23. Kirk VG, Clausen MM, Armitage MD, et al. Preverbal photoscreening for amblyogenic factors and outcomes in amblyopia treatment: early objective screening and visual acuities. Arch Ophthalmol 2008;126(4):489–92.
24. Vision screening recommendations. AAPOS Web site. Copyright 2014. Available at: www.aapos.org/ahp/vision_screening_recommendations/. Accessed January 30, 2014.

Amblyopia

Diana DeSantis, MD

KEYWORDS

- Amblyopia • Atropine • Levodopa • Patching

KEY POINTS

- Amblyopia is the most common cause of vision loss in children.
- Early detection and treatment of amblyopia are critical to restoring vision in amblyopic eyes.
- Regular vision screening and appropriate referral to a pediatric ophthalmologist are important steps in the detection of children at risk for amblyopia.
- The Pediatric Eye Disease Investigator Group (PEDIG) has published several studies in recent years providing evidence on which to base treatment decisions. Newer treatments including atropine drops and oral levodopa have been evaluated.

With an estimated prevalence of 2% to 4% in North America, amblyopia accounts for more cases of unilateral reduced vision in children than all other causes combined.[1] By definition, amblyopia refers to unilateral or, less commonly, bilateral reduction in best corrected visual acuity, not directly attributed to a structural abnormality of the eye or posterior visual pathways.[1] Its primary causes are strabismus, anisometropia (significant difference in refractive error between the 2 eyes) or bilateral high refractive errors, and stimulus deprivation. Early detection of amblyopia is crucial in obtaining the best response to treatment. If amblyopia goes unrecognized or untreated past the early years of life, it often cannot be successfully treated and vision cannot be fully restored in the amblyopic eye. Although there are exceptions to the rule, most ophthalmologists regard the age of visual maturity to be approximately 8 to 9 years of age. Beyond visual maturity, most cases of amblyopia respond poorly to any form of treatment. It is also generally accepted that amblyopia responds best to treatment in the first few years of life.

The earliest clinical description of human amblyopia is generally credited to Le Cat in 1713. Although amblyopia as a disease has been relatively well understood for many years and the treatment modalities have remained fairly standard, in the past several years much has been published regarding this disease, owing mostly to a series of Amblyopia Treatment Studies (ATS) undertaken by the Pediatric Eye Disease Investigator Group (PEDIG). These studies were designed to evaluate the traditional methods for treating amblyopia and provide evidence on which to base treatment decisions.

Children's Eye Physicians, 4875 Ward Road, Wheat Ridge, CO 80033, USA
E-mail address: ddesantis@cepcolorado.com

Pediatr Clin N Am 61 (2014) 505–518
http://dx.doi.org/10.1016/j.pcl.2014.03.006
0031-3955/14/$ – see front matter © 2014 Elsevier Inc. All rights reserved.
pediatric.theclinics.com

Before the PEDIG studies, most published studies on amblyopia treatment were large retrospective reviews.[2]

Formed in 1997, and funded by the National Eye Institute, PEDIG is a collaborative network facilitating multicenter clinical research in strabismus, amblyopia, and other eye disorders that affect children. There are more than 100 participating sites with more than 200 pediatric ophthalmologists and optometrists in the United States, Canada, and the United Kingdom. PEDIG has completed more than 15 ATS to date, many with multiple phases. The published findings of the PEDIG ATS to date are summarized in **Table 1**.

As presented as part of a 2006 Symposium at the Joint Meeting of the American Orthoptic Council, the American Association of Certified Orthoptists, and the American Academy of Ophthalmology, and subsequently reported in the *American Orthoptic Journal* in 2007, David K. Wallace has summarized several questions regarding amblyopia and its treatment that have been addressed by the PEDIG studies, including the following:

1. How well do glasses alone treat amblyopia?
2. Do we really know that patching works?
3. How many daily hours of prescribed patching are necessary?
4. What happens when patching is stopped?
5. Does patching work in older children?
6. Does atropine work as well as patching?
7. How often does atropine need to be used?
8. If improvement plateaus with patching, is it beneficial to increase patching time?

The following discussion summarizes the findings of the various PEDIG studies as they relate to these questions.

HOW WELL DO GLASSES ALONE TREAT AMBLYOPIA?

This question was the subject of the spectacle phase of ATS 5. Eighty-four patients participated, ranging in age from 3 to 7 years. Follow-up was up to 30 weeks. The results of this study demonstrated that 77% of amblyopic eyes improved by 2 or more lines of vision by using optical correction alone. Resolution of amblyopia using optical correction alone occurred in 27% of patients.[3]

DO WE REALLY KNOW THAT PATCHING WORKS?

This question was the subject of the ATS 5 randomized clinical trial phase. A total of 180 patients, ranging in age from 3 to 7 years, were followed for 5 weeks. After no further vision improvement with glasses alone, these patients were treated with 2 hours per day of patching combined with 1 hour of near visual tasks. In this group of patients, vision improved 1.1 lines compared with 0.5 lines in a control group.[4]

HOW MANY DAILY HOURS OF PRESCRIBED PATCHING ARE NECESSARY?

ATS 2A compared full-time with 6 hours of daily patching for those with visual acuity 20/100 to 20/400. A total of 175 patients between the ages of 3 and 7 years participated, with a follow-up of 4 months. In these patients, the vision improved 4.8 lines in the group patching 6 hours per day and 4.7 lines in the group patching full time. ATS 2B compared 6 hours of daily patching with 2 hours of patching per day for those with visual acuities ranging from 20/40 to 20/80. A total of 189 patients ranging in age from 3 to 7 years were studied, with a follow-up of 4 months. The improvement of

Table 1
Pediatric Eye Disease Investigator Group studies with published results

Study	No. of Patients (Age at Enrollment)	Follow-Up Period	Result
Randomized trial comparing occlusion vs pharmacologic for moderate amblyopia (ATS 1)	419 (3 to <7 y)	6 mo	VA improved in both groups: 3.16 lines in occlusion group; 2.84 lines in atropine group Mean difference = 0.34 lines (95% CI, 0.05–0.6) VA ≥20/30 and/or improved by ≥3 lines in 79% of occlusion group and 74% of atropine group
Randomized trial comparing occlusion vs pharmacologic therapy for moderate amblyopia (ATS 1)	419 (3 to <7 y)	2 y	VA improved in both groups: 3.7 lines in occlusion group; 3.6 lines in atropine group Mean difference = 0.01 lines (95% CI, −0.02 to 0.04) Atropine or patching for an initial 6-mo period produced a similar improvement in amblyopia 2 y after treatment
Randomized trial comparing part-time vs full-time patching for severe amblyopia (ATS 2A)	175 (3 to <7 y)	4 mo	VA improved in both groups: 4.8 lines in the 6-h patching group; 4.7 lines in the full-time patching (all hours or all but 1 h per day) group Mean difference = 0.02 lines (95% CI, −0.04 to 0.07)
Randomized trial comparing part-time vs minimal-time patching for moderate amblyopia (ATS 2B)	189 (3 to <7 y)	4 mo	VA improvement in both groups was 2.40 lines Mean difference = −0.007 lines (95% CI, −0.050 to 0.036) VA ≥20/32 and/or ≥3 lines in 62% of patients in both groups VA improvement similar for 2 h of daily patching and 6 h of daily patching

(continued on next page)

Table 1
(continued)

Study	No. of Patients (Age at Enrollment)	Follow-Up Period	Result
Evaluation of treatment of amblyopia (ATS 3)	507 (7–17 y)	6 mo	For moderate amblyopia in children 7 to <13 y old, 36% achieved 20/25 or better with optical correction/occlusion/atropine use compared with 14% with optical correction alone ($P<.001$)
			For severe amblyopia in children 7 to <13 y old, 23% achieved 20/40 or better with optical correction/patching compared with 5% with optical correction alone ($P<.004$)
			For moderate amblyopia in teenagers 13–17 y old, 14% achieved 20/25 or better with optical correction/occlusion compared with 11% with optical correction alone ($P = .52$)
			For severe amblyopia in teenagers 13–17 y old, 14% achieved 20/25 or better with optical correction/occlusion compared with 0% with optical correction alone ($P = .13$)
Randomized trial comparing daily atropine vs weekend atropine for moderate amblyopia (ATS 4)	168 (3 to <7 y)	4 mo	VA improvement in both groups was 2.3 lines Mean difference = 0.00 (95% CI, −0.04 to 0.04) 47% of daily group and 53% of the weekend group had either VA ≥20/25 or greater than or equal to that of the nonamblyopic eye
Prospective noncomparative trial to evaluate 2 h of daily patching for amblyopia (ATS 5, eyeglasses-only phase)	84 (3 to <7 y)	Up to 30 wk	Amblyopia improved with optical correction by ≥2 lines in 77% Amblyopia resolved with optical correction in 27% (95% CI, 18%–38%)

Randomized trial to evaluate 2 h daily patching for amblyopia (ATS 5, randomization phase)	180 (3 to <7 y)	5 wk	After a period of treatment with eyeglasses until vision stopped improving, patients treated with 2 h of daily patching combined with 1 h of near visual tasks had an improvement in VA of 1.1 lines compared with 0.5 lines in the control group Mean difference (adjusted) = 0.07 lines (95% CI, 0.02–0.12; P = .006)
Randomized trial to compare near vs distance activities while occluded (ATS 6)	425 (3 to <7 y)	17 wk	At 8 wk, improvement in amblyopic eye VA averaged 2.6 lines in the distance activities group and 2.5 lines in the near activities group (95% CI for difference, −0.3 to 0.3 line) Groups appeared statistically similar at the 2-wk, 5-wk, and 17-wk visits At 17 wk, children with severe amblyopia improved a mean of 3.7 lines with 2 h patching
Treatments of bilateral refractive amblyopia (ATS 7)	113 (3 to <10 y)	1 y	Binocular VA improved on average 3.9 lines (95% CI, 3.5–4.2) At 1 y, 74% had binocular VA of 20/25 or better
Randomized trial comparing atropine vs atropine plus a plano lens for the fellow eye in children 3–6 y (ATS 8)	180 (3 to <7 y)	18 wk	Amblyopic eye VA was 20/25 or better in 29% of the atropine-only group and in 40% of the atropine plus plano lens group (P = .03) More patients in the atropine plus plano lens group had reduced fellow eye acuity at 18 wk; however, there were no cases of persistent reverse amblyopia
Randomized trial comparing occlusion vs atropine for amblyopia (ATS 9)	193 (7 to <13 y)	17 wk	Similar improvement in VA in both groups Amblyopic eye VA of 20/25 or better in 17% of atropine group and 24% of the patching group (95% CI, −3% to 17%)

(continued on next page)

Table 1 (*continued*)			
Study	**No. of Patients (Age at Enrollment)**	**Follow-Up Period**	**Result**
Randomized trial comparing Bangerter filters vs occlusion for the treatment of moderate amblyopia in children (ATS 10)	186 (3 to <10 y)	24 wk	Similar improvement in VA in both groups Amblyopic eye VA of 20/25 or better in 36% of Bangerter group and 31% of patching group (*P* = .86) Patching was not superior (95% CI difference between groups, −0.06 to 0.83 line)
Randomized trial to evaluate combined patching and atropine for residual amblyopia (ATS 11)	55 (3 to <10 y)	10 wk	Before enrollment, eligible subjects had no improvement with 6 h daily patching or daily atropine Intensive treatment group had 6 h of prescribed daily patching combined with daily atropine; weaning group had 4 wk of reduced treatment, then stopped Amblyopic eye VA improved similarly in both groups, an average of 0.56 lines in the intensive group (95% CI, 0.18–0.93) and 0.53 lines in the weaning group (95% CI, −0.04 to 1.10)
Nonrandomized prospective trial of eyeglasses alone for strabismic and strabismic-anisometropic combined amblyopia in children (ATS 13)	146 (3 to <7 y)	28 wk	Mean 2.6 lines improvement (95% CI, 2.3–3.0) 75% improved ≥2 lines and 54% improved ≥3 lines Resolution in 32% (95% CI, 24%–41%) Treatment effect was greater for combined-mechanism amblyopia (3.2 vs 2.3 lines; adjusted *P* = .003)

In the ATS, mild to moderate amblyopia is defined as VA in the amblyopic eye of 20/80 or better; severe amblyopia is defined as VA in the amblyopic eye of 20/100 to 20/400.

Further information about the published results of the Amblyopia Treatment Study is available from the Pediatric Eye Disease Investigator Group (http://pedig.jaeb.org/Publications.aspx).

Abbreviations: ATS, amblyopia treatment study; CI, confidence interval; VA, visual acuity.

From American Academy of Ophthalmology Pediatric Ophthalmology/Strabismus Panel. Preferred Practice Pattern ® Guidelines. Amblyopia. San Francisco (CA): American Academy of Ophthalmology; 2012. Available at: www.aao.org/ppp; with permission.

visual acuity was 2.4 lines in both groups, indicating that 2 hours of daily patching can be equally as effective as 6 hours per day.[5,6]

WHAT HAPPENS WHEN PATCHING STOPS?

ATS 2C studied 156 patients with either strabismic or anisometropic amblyopia. These patients had been treated at least 3 months with 2 or more hours of daily patching or once-weekly atropine, and had achieved at least 3 lines of visual improvement. Patients were examined at 5, 13, 26, and 52 weeks following cessation of patching or atropine. Recurrence occurred in 21% patients at 1 year. Most recurrences occurred in the first 5 weeks after stopping treatment. Those with intense patching (6–8 hours per day) had more recurrence if weaning did not occur.[7]

DOES PATCHING WORK IN OLDER CHILDREN?

ATS 3 evaluated 507 patients between the ages of 7 and 17 years. Patients were randomized to optical correction alone versus optical correction plus patching. Patients under the age of 13 also used atropine. After 6 months of follow-up, patching plus atropine was found to be superior to glasses alone in patients aged 7 to 12 years. In the 13- to 17-year-old age group, there was no significant difference between optical correction alone and optical correction plus patching, unless the patient had received no previous treatment.[8]

DOES ATROPINE WORK AS WELL AS PATCHING?

ATS 1 was a randomized clinical trial of patching versus atropine as primary treatment of moderate amblyopia, defined by this study as baseline amblyopic eye visual acuity 20/40 to 20/100. A total of 419 patients between the ages of 3 and 7 years were followed at 6 months and again at 2 years. Both groups improved approximately 3 lines in visual acuity, and sensory outcomes at 2 years were also similar.[9,10]

HOW OFTEN DOES ATROPINE NEED TO BE USED?

ATS 4 followed 168 patients aged 3 to 7 years for 4 months, comparing daily atropine with weekend-only atropine for moderate amblyopia with acuities ranging from 20/40 to 20/80. In these patients, the improvement in visual acuity was 2.3 lines in both groups, and stereoacuity outcomes were similar.[11]

The most recently published PEDIG study results compare the effectiveness of increasing hours of patching from 2 to 6 hours per day in children with stable residual amblyopia. A total of 168 patients between the ages of 3 and 8 years participated. Patients had been patching 2 hours per day for 12 weeks and were randomized to either continue 2 hours patching per day or increase to 6 hours per day for 10 weeks. In these patients the 6 hours per day group improved an average of 1.2 lines, with 40% improving 2 lines or more. The 2 hours per day group improved an average of 0.5 lines, with 19% improving 2 lines or more.[12]

L-DOPA IN THE TREATMENT OF AMBLYOPIA

A key aspect to the understanding of amblyopia is that it is considered a brain problem rather than an eye problem. Parents often find this somewhat confusing, because amblyopia is often referred to by the lay term "lazy eye." It is best if physicians and eye-care professionals refrain from using this term, because it also often implies strabismus or ptosis, and the treatment of these conditions is very different. Much of what is known about the anatomic and physiologic properties of visual cortical cells, which provide the foundation to understanding the pathophysiology of amblyopia, was established by the scientific research of David Hubel and Torsten Wiesel, for which they were awarded the 1981 Nobel Prize in Medicine.[13–17] Based on the work of Hubel and Wiesel, it is believed that amblyopia results when one eye takes control of most visual cortical cells. Binocular competition depends on age, which is why there is a "critical" or "plastic" time in a child's life when amblyopia therapy is effective.

The critical period of visual development is not only affected by age but also by the presence of certain neurotransmitters and neuromodulators in the brain.[18–20] Kasamatsu and Pettigrew[19] provided scientific evidence for the hypothesis that dopaminergic drugs may influence the plasticity and recovery of vision in the amblyopic eye. This discovery led to a new approach to amblyopia therapy. Instead of penalization therapy to the sound eye, pharmacologic therapy to improve the vision in the amblyopic eye is now being considered as a treatment for amblyopia that has failed traditional treatments. Treatment failure can result from late age of detection, poor compliance with prescribed treatment, and severity of visual loss or density of amblyopia.

Gottlob and Stangler-Zuschrott[21,22] were the first to evaluate the effects of the dopamine precursor levodopa in adults with amblyopia. Since they first published their work in 1990, Leguire and colleagues[23–27] have investigated the use of levodopa/carbidopa, the dosage of medication, concomitant use of patching, and recidivism of visual gains. Their results support the hypothesis that treatment with L-dopa plus occlusion improves vision and provides a lasting improvement in the vision of amblyopic eyes that have failed traditional therapy. These studies along with others[28–31] have provided the foundation for the current PEDIG study, ATS 17. This study prospectively looks at the visual improvement in eyes that have failed or plateaued with traditional therapy. Also evaluated in this study is the use of concomitant patching. One arm of ATS 17 included the use of placebo drug with the expectation that results will add significant information about the use of L-dopa therapy for amblyopia. This study is now closed and the results are pending.

SCREENING FOR AMBLYOPIA

The key to early detection of amblyopia is vision screening, which begins in the first 6 months of life by the assessment of fixation and following response or tracking of objects. According to the recommendations of the American Association for Pediatric Ophthalmology and Strabismus (AAPOS), infants who do not display good tracking and those with an abnormality of the red reflex should be referred for a formal eye examination,[32] preferably to a pediatric ophthalmologist.

From 6 months until a child is capable of reading a vision-testing chart, vision screening may be assessed using an automated screening device such as a photoscreener, which uses the red reflex to identify many types of ocular problems. Children who are identified as having a potential eye problem by photoscreening, in addition to those with strabismus or an abnormal red reflex, should be referred for a complete eye examination.

After the age of 3 or 4 years, most children are able to cooperate with vision testing using a Snellen eye chart. There are many options for the testing of preliterate children, such as Allen figures, tumbling E charts, and HOTV charts. Children younger than 5 years should be able to identify most of the figures on the 20/40 line with either eye individually. Those who are unable to see the 20/40 line with either eye should be referred for ophthalmologic examination according to AAPOS guidelines.[32]

After the age of 5 years, most children should be capable of seeing most of the figures on the 20/30 line of an eye chart, and those who are unable to do so should be referred. Screening should be repeated every 1 to 2 years during the elementary school years.[32]

The necessity for a formal eye examination for all children before the start of kindergarten remains a subject of debate, with most pediatric ophthalmologists adopting the position that screening may be successfully accomplished by primary care physicians and through school screenings. **Table 2**, from www.aapos.org, outlines the AAPOS

Table 2
American Association for Pediatric Ophthalmology and Strabismus vision screening recommendations

Age	Tests	Referral Criteria Comments
Newborn to 6 mo	Ocular history Vision assessment External inspection of the eyes and lids Ocular motility assessment Pupil examination Red reflex examination	Refer infants who do not track well after 3 mo of age Refer infants with an abnormal red reflex or history of retinoblastoma in a parent or sibling
6–42 mo	Ocular history Vision assessment External inspection of the eyes and lids Ocular motility assessment Pupil examination Red reflex examination Visual acuity testing Objective screening device photoscreening Ophthalmoscopy	Refer infants with strabismus Refer infants with chronic tearing or discharge Refer children who fail photoscreening
42 mo to 5 y	Ocular history Vision assessment External inspection of the eyes and lids Ocular motility assessment Pupil examination Red reflex examination Visual acuity testing (preferred) or photoscreening Ophthalmoscopy	Refer children who cannot read at least 20/40 with either eye. Must be able to identify most of the optotypes on the 20/40 line Refer children who fail photoscreening
≥5 y[a]	Ocular history Vision assessment External inspection of the eyes and lids Ocular motility assessment Pupil examination Red reflex examination Visual acuity testing Ophthalmoscopy	Refer children who cannot read at least 20/32 with either eye. Must be able to identify most of the optotypes on the 20/32 line Refer children not reading at grade level

[a] Repeat screening every 1–2 y or after age 5.
From American Association for Pediatric Ophthalmology and Strabismus (AAPOS). Available at: http://www.aapos.org/terms/conditions/131.

guidelines for vision screening and referral recommendations for children at various ages.[32]

CLASSIFICATION

Most cases of amblyopia can be classified as strabismic, anisometropic, ametropic, or stimulus deprivation. Strabismic amblyopia typically is the result of a constant, nonalternating or unequally alternating manifest misalignment of the eyes.[33] Amblyopia is much more likely to occur with acquired or accommodative esotropia than with either congenital esotropia or intermittent exotropia. In addition to treating the amblyopia itself, these patients also require correction of the underlying strabismus using glasses or other refractive correction, along with surgical intervention when the remaining ocular misalignment is significant enough to prevent maintenance of vision in both eyes.

Anisometropic amblyopia develops when unequal refractive error in the two eyes causes the image on one retina to be chronically more defocused than that of the fellow eye.[33] Amblyopia can occur with as little as one diopter difference in hyperopia between the two eyes, usually occurring in the more hyperopic eye. In patients with myopic refractive errors, higher degrees of anisometropia can be tolerated without leading to the development of amblyopia. Myopic anisometropia of 3 diopters or less typically does not result in the development of amblyopia. However, unilateral high myopia of 6 diopters or more often results in severe amblyopia.[1] In the case of hyperopic or astigmatic anisometropia, amblyopia may result from relatively minor differences of 1 to 2 diopters between the two eyes.[1]

Ametropic amblyopia may occur in both eyes with bilateral high refractive errors on the order of 6 or more diopters of myopia, 5 or more diopters of hyperopia, or 2 or greater diopters of astigmatism.[1]

Stimulus deprivation amblyopia most commonly occurs as a result of complete or partial obstruction of the visual axis during the early critical period of vision development. The most common cause is congenital cataract, but deprivation amblyopia can also result from severe congenital ptosis, corneal opacity, or an orbital lesion such as a hemangioma affecting the visual axis. The period of time required for deprivational amblyopia to occur is much shorter than that of strabismic or anisometropic amblyopia, and deprivation amblyopia generally occurs much earlier in life than the other types of amblyopia. Visual deprivation in the early months of life is strongly associated with the development of sensory nystagmus and strabismus.[33]

DIAGNOSIS

The initial amblyopia evaluation should include a complete ophthalmic examination with attention to risk factors for amblyopia such as strabismus, anisometropia, media opacity, or other structural defects, as well as positive family history for strabismus or amblyopia. Cycloplegia (dilation) is necessary for obtaining an accurate refraction. The diagnosis of amblyopia may be made when the affected eye cannot be corrected to 20/20 or there is a 2 or greater line difference in visual acuity between the two eyes. In preverbal children, the diagnosis can be made if there is asymmetric objection to occlusion of one eye or failure to maintain fixation with one eye. In cases of bilateral amblyopia, the diagnosis is suspected if the best corrected visual acuity in either eye measures worse than 20/50 in children 3 years of age or younger, or worse than 20/40 in a child older than 4 years.[33] Amblyopic eyes frequently display what is known as the crowding phenomenon, which refers to the worsening of Snellen acuities when presented with a row of images on the eye chart as opposed to isolated individual figures.

TREATMENT

Success rates of amblyopia treatment decline with increasing age.[33] Treatment should consist of the elimination of any obstacle to vision, correction of significant refractive errors, and forced use of the amblyopic eye by occluding fellow eye.

In children with deprivation amblyopia, the initial treatment should be directed at removing the obstruction of the visual axis. Congenital cataracts that are visually significant should be removed as quickly as possible to prevent visual deprivation, and appropriate aphakic optical correction should be in place as promptly as is feasible following removal of the cataract. Aphakic optical correction may be achieved using intraocular lens implants in children who are deemed appropriate candidates, contact lenses, or aphakic spectacles. In some cases, a combination of these methods of optical correction may be necessary.

Optical correction in children with anisometropic or refractive amblyopia is usually achieved by the use of eyeglasses. Recent studies have shown that treatment of refractive error alone can substantially improve visual acuity in eyes with amblyopia.[3]

When optical correction alone does not result in normal vision in an amblyopic eye, occlusion of the sound eye is often required. The use of an orthoptic eye patch remains the gold standard for occlusion therapy. For children who cannot tolerate a patch there are alternative methods, such as the use of an occlusive contact lens on the sound eye or the use of a Bangerter filter over the glasses lens of the eye to be occluded. There are a variety of densities of filter available, depending on the level of optical degradation required.

Pharmacologic penalization may be used as an alternative or adjunct to patching if the sound eye is hyperopic. Atropine 1% ophthalmic solution is typically used to cause cycloplegia in the sound eye, resulting in an optically defocused image. This approach may be used in children with mild to moderate amblyopia. Atropine may also be used in conjunction with optical penalization, which typically refers to reducing the hyperopic correction in the sound eye or replacing the lens of the sound eye with a plano (clear) lens temporarily. There have been reports of transient reduction of visual acuity in the nonamblyopic eye resulting from the use of atropine, particularly when used in combination with reduced hyperopic correction.[33] Photosensitivity may also result from the use of atropine, particularly in areas of high sun exposure.[33] Systemic adverse effects may include dryness of the mouth, tachycardia, fever, and delirium.[33]

In addition to the previously discussed treatment modalities, the American Academy of Ophthalmology Preferred Practice Patterns guidelines for amblyopia treatment include controversial or alternative therapies such as refractive surgery, acupuncture, and vision therapy.

The role of refractive surgery in the treatment of anisometropic amblyopia remains controversial. Some studies have shown keratorefractive surgery to be a safe procedure in children with anisometropic amblyopia who are noncompliant with refractive correction.[33] At present, keratorefractive surgery in children is an off-label use of an FDA-approved device. Refractive procedures may have a future role in the management of amblyopia in certain children who fail conventional treatment.[33]

Acupuncture in the treatment of amblyopia has been studied in limited clinical trials. These studies have reported acupuncture to be effective in the treatment of amblyopia, both as an alternative to occlusion therapy and as an adjunct to refractive correction. The mechanism of action for acupuncture in the treatment of amblyopia is unknown, and further investigation is required.[33]

Vision therapy has also been promoted by some in the treatment of amblyopia, as primary therapy or as an adjunct or alternative to patching. Vision therapy may take various forms, depending on the eye-care professional, including muscle exercises, pursuit or tracking exercises, and glasses with or without bifocals or prisms. Although vision therapy has been in use by some eye-care professionals for many years, there are to date insufficient cohort studies or randomized clinical trials to support the use of these techniques.[33]

COMPLICATIONS

Potential complications of amblyopia treatment include the possibility of inducing occlusion amblyopia in the previously sound eye when using an occlusive patch. Infants and very young children are more sensitive to occlusion, and therefore should be checked at regular intervals to monitor for the development of occlusion amblyopia in the previously sound eye. The period of time between the initiation of patching and the follow-up evaluation should be tailored to the age of the patient and the severity of the amblyopia. Fortunately, occlusion amblyopia can typically be reversed if recognized and treated promptly. Another possible complication of amblyopia treatment is the development of manifest strabismus that was either not manifest or not present before initiation of amblyopia treatment. This complication has been described with patching treatment, particularly full-time occlusion, use of full optical correction, and use of pharmacologic or optical penalization. Another potential pitfall associated with amblyopia treatment is that of poor compliance with prescribed treatment, particularly with patching therapy and in children with very dense amblyopia. In addition, anisometropic children with excellent uncorrected vision in the sound eye may resist full-time use of glasses.

If a patient fails to respond to treatment, despite apparent good compliance with glasses and patching, it may be helpful to change the method of treatment or to introduce something new, such as atropine with or without optical penalization.

Recurrence of amblyopia is not uncommon following cessation of treatment. Often the vision will stabilize 1 or 2 lines below the best visual acuity achieved while the patient was actively patching. Recurrence of amblyopia may be avoided or limited by avoiding discontinuing treatment prematurely, by weaning patching as opposed to abruptly discontinuing patching, and by following patients closely after discontinuation of the patch or other treatment.

SUMMARY

Amblyopia is the most common cause of preventable vision loss in children. With early detection, amblyopia can be successfully treated and normal vision restored. Early detection relies on appropriate vision screening, starting in the first few months of life and continuing at regular intervals in the early years of life. Prompt referral for a formal complete eye examination following failed screening is crucial for the diagnosis of amblyopia, treatment of the underlying cause, and initiation of occlusion or other treatment. The amblyopia treatment studies carried out by PEDIG have recently provided an evidence basis for the various types of treatment used.

REFERENCES

1. Raab EL. Amblyopia. In: Raab EL, editor. Basic and Clinical Science Course 2010–2011 Section 6: Pediatric Ophthalmology and Strabismus. San Francisco (CA): American Academy of Ophthalmology; 2010. p. 61–9.
2. Wallace DK. Evidence-based amblyopia treatment: results of PEDIG studies. Am Orthopt J 2007;57:48–55.

3. Cotter SA, Pediatric Eye Disease Investigator Group, Edwards AR, et al. Treatment of anisometropic amblyopia in children with refractive correction. Ophthalmology 2006;113:895–903.
4. Wallace DK, Pediatric Eye Disease Investigator Group, Edwards AR, et al. A randomized trial to evaluate 2 hours of daily patching for strabismic and anisometropic amblyopia in children. Ophthalmology 2006;113:904–12.
5. Pediatric Eye Disease Investigator Group, Holmes JM, Kraker RT, et al. A randomized trial of prescribed patching regimens for treatment of severe amblyopia in children. Ophthalmology 2003;110:2075–87.
6. Pediatric Eye Disease Investigator Group, Repka MX, Beck RW, et al. A randomized trial of patching regimens for treatment of moderate amblyopia in children. Arch Ophthalmol 2003;121:603–11.
7. Pediatric Eye Disease Investigator Group, Holmes JM, Beck RW, et al. Risk of amblyopia recurrence after cessation of treatment. J AAPOS 2004;8:420–8.
8. Pediatric Eye Disease Investigator Group, Scheiman MM, Hertle RW, et al. Randomized trial of treatment of amblyopia in children aged 7 to 17 years. Arch Ophthalmol 2005;123:437–47.
9. Pediatric Eye Disease Investigator Group. A randomized trial of atropine vs. patching for treatment of moderate amblyopia in children. Arch Ophthalmol 2002;120:268–78.
10. Pediatric Eye Disease Investigator Group, Repka MX, Wallace DK, et al. Two-year follow-up of a 6-month randomized trial of atropine vs. patching for treatment of moderate amblyopia in children. Arch Ophthalmol 2005;123:149–57.
11. Pediatric Eye Disease Investigator Group, Repka MX, Cotter SA, et al. A randomized trial of atropine regimens for treatment of moderate amblyopia in children. Ophthalmology 2004;111:2076–85.
12. Pediatric Eye Disease Investigator Group, Wallace DK, Lazar EL, et al. A randomized trial of increasing patching for amblyopia. Ophthalmology 2013; 120:2270–7.
13. Wiesel TN, Hubel DH. Single cell responses in striate cortex of kittens deprived of vision in one eye. J Neurophysiol 1963;26:1003–17.
14. Hubel DH, Weisel TN. Functional architecture of macaque monkey visual cortex. Proc R Soc Lond B Biol Sci 1977;28(198):1–59.
15. Hubel DH, Wiesel TN, LeVay S. Plasticity of ocular dominance columns in monkey striate cortex. Philos Trans R Soc Lond B Biol Sci 1977;278:377–409.
16. LeVay S, Wiesel TN, Hubel DH. The development of ocular dominance columns in normal and visually deprived monkeys. J Comp Neurol 1980;19:1–51.
17. Wiesel TN. Postnatal development of the visual cortex and the influence of environment. Nature 1982;299:583–91.
18. Kasamatsu T, Pettigrew JD, Ary M. Restoration of visual cortical plasticity by local microperfusion of norepinephrine. J Comp Neurol 1979;185:168–81.
19. Kasamatsu T, Pettigrew JD. Preservation of binocularity after monocular deprivation in the striate cortex of kittens treated with 6-hydroxydopamine. J Comp Neurol 1979;185:139–61.
20. Imamura K, Kasamatsu LK, Nairus TM, et al. Long-term follow-up of L-DOPA treatment in children with amblyopia. J Pediatr Ophthalmol Strabismus 2002;39:326–30.
21. Gottlob I, Strangler-Zuschrott E. Effect of levodopa on contrast sensitivity and scotomas in human amblyopia. Invest Ophthalmol Vis Sci 1990;31:776–80.
22. Gottlob I, Charlier J, Reinecke RD. Visual acuities and scotomas after one-week levodopa administration in human amblyopia. Invest Ophthalmol Vis Sci 1992;33: 2722–8.

23. Leguire LE, Rogers GL, Walson PD, et al. Occlusion and levodopa-carbidopa treatment for childhood amblyopia. J AAPOS 1998;2:257–64.
24. Leguire LE, Rogers GL, Bremer DL, et al. Levodopa and childhood amblyopia. J Pediatr Ophthalmol Strabismus 1992;29:290–8.
25. Leguire LE, Rogers GL, Bremer DL, et al. Levodopa/carbidopa for childhood amblyopia. Invest Ophthalmol Vis Sci 1993;34:3090–5.
26. Leguire LE, Walson PD, Rogers GL, et al. Longitudinal study of levodopa/carbidopa for childhood amblyopia. J Pediatr Ophthalmol Strabismus 1993;30: 354–60.
27. Leguire LE, Walson PD, Rogers GL, et al. Levodopa/carbidopa treatment for amblyopia in older children. J Pediatr Ophthalmol Strabismus 1995;32:143–51.
28. Gottlob I, Wizov SS, Reinecke RD. Visual acuities and scotomas after 3 weeks' levodopa administration in adult amblyopia. Graefes Arch Clin Exp Ophthalmol 1995;233(7):407–13.
29. Mohan K, Dhankar V, Sharma A. Visual acuities after levodopa administration in amblyopia. J Pediatr Ophthalmol Strabismus 2001;38(2):62–7.
30. Procianoy E, Fuchs FD, Procianoy L, et al. The effect of increasing doses of levodopa on children with strabismic amblyopia. J AAPOS 1999;3(6):337–40.
31. Bhartiya P, Sharma P, Biswas NR, et al. Levodopa-carbidopa with occlusion in older children with amblyopia. J AAPOS 2002;6(6):368–72.
32. Patient Info. Vision screening recommendations. Available at: http://www.aapos.org/terms.
33. American Academy of Ophthalmology Pediatric Ophthalmology/Strabismus Panel. Preferred practice pattern® guidelines. Amblyopia. San Francisco (CA): American Academy of Ophthalmology; 2012. Available at: www.aao.org/ppp.

Pediatric Refractive Surgery

Erin D. Stahl, MD[a,b,*]

KEYWORDS

- Refractive surgery • Pediatrics • Photorefractive keratectomy • LASIK
- Phakic intraocular lens

KEY POINTS

- Pediatric refractive surgery has different indications than adult refractive surgery.
- Refractive surgery is for children who are failing with cognitive or visual development because of refractive error.
- There are many surgical options for pediatric refractive surgery patients.
- Challenges with pediatric refractive surgery include logistics, patient cooperation, anesthesia, high refractive errors, and amblyopia.
- Pediatric refractive surgery includes off-label treatments.

INTRODUCTION

Refractive surgery, or surgery to eliminate the need for eyeglasses or contact lenses, has become a common and well-accepted elective surgery across the world. Adult refractive surgery is an environment with rapidly changing technology, techniques, and vast advances over the past 40 years. With greater experience of refractive surgery in the adult population, the pediatric community has begun to show special interest in using these techniques to help a new population of patients. As pediatric clinicians proceed into the realm of refractive surgery, additional challenges, adaptations, and concerns about this emerging practice arise. Careful consideration of the unique aspects of visual development combined with lessons learned during the history of adult refractive surgery are joined to offer children novel and effective therapies for treating select conditions.

HISTORICAL PERSPECTIVE

Modern refractive surgery started in 1950 with Columbian ophthalmologist Jose Barraquer and his development of an instrument to create a corneal flap for the purpose of correcting refractive errors termed "keratomileusis." In 1974 radial keratotomy, which

[a] Pediatric Ophthalmology, University of Missouri-Kansas City, Kansas City, MO 64108, USA;
[b] Department of Ophthalmology, University of Kansas, Prairie Village, KS 66206, USA
* Children's Mercy Hospitals and Clinics, 2401 Gillham Road, Kansas City, MO 64108.
E-mail address: edstahl@cmh.edu

Pediatr Clin N Am 61 (2014) 519–527
http://dx.doi.org/10.1016/j.pcl.2014.03.008 **pediatric.theclinics.com**

consists of making radial partial-thickness cuts in the cornea, was introduced by Svyatoslav Fyodorov for the treatment of myopia. Excimer laser was first proposed for the treatment of corneal refractive errors by US ophthalmologist Stephen Trokel in 1983.[1] Laser technology evolved rapidly and photorefractive keratectomy (PRK) was first performed on humans in the mid-1980s by Theo Seiler. As a melding of PRK and Barraquer's early thoughts on keratomileusis, laser-assisted in situ kerato-mileusis (LASIK) was first performed in 1990 by Lucio Burrato and Ioannis Pallikaris.

When the first lasers were introduced the obvious initial candidates for treatment were those with large, often debilitating refractive errors. After initial success with the treatment of high refractive errors, clinicians began to note complications with haze, excessive corneal thinning, and scarring in some patients.[2–4] Researchers began to look for alternative technology for the treatment of high refractive errors and reserved laser technology for low-to-moderate refractive errors.

The first phakic intraocular lens (PIOL) was implanted in 1990 for the treatment of high myopia.[5] This surgery placed the PIOL in the anterior chamber without disruption of the crystalline lens. Further studies have shown that the PIOL technologies provided excellent optical outcomes in patients with high refractive errors.[6–8] Because this technology is more invasive than surface refractive procedures, risks include endothe-lial cell damage, cataract formation, risk for retinal detachment, and the generally increased risk of intraocular surgery.[9,10]

Another treatment modality that has evolved for large refractive errors is lensectomy with or without implantation of a low-power or plano IOL.[11] This technique, termed "refractive lens exchange," has been used for patients with large refractive errors and adult patients desiring multifocal IOLs to treat presbyopia and refractive error in one procedure (**Boxes 1** and **2**).

REFRACTIVE SURGERY PROCEDURES TODAY IN ADULTS
Low-to-moderate Myopia and Low Hyperopia

After determination that the patient is a suitable candidate for refractive surgery (adequate corneal thickness, normal corneal architecture, absence of other pathology, realistic expectations, and stability of current refractive error) most of these low-to-moderate myopes and hyperopes are excellent excimer laser candidates. Generally, laser correction (either LASIK or PRK) is the procedure of choice for refractions ranging from approximately +3.00 diopter (D) to −8.00 D, depending on many factors identified in the preoperative visit. This is the range where the author finds maximization of refrac-tive outcomes, stability, and patient satisfaction with excimer laser surgery.

High Myopia

Decisions about treatment options for moderate-to-high myopia often hinge on age and refractive error. In young patients with greater than −8.00 D of myopia, laser

---

Box 1
Historical timeline of refractive surgery treatments

1950 – Keratomileusis

1974 – Radial keratotomy to treat myopia

1983 – PRK using an excimer laser

1990 – LASIK using an excimer laser

1990 – PIOL

Box 2
List of refractive eye surgery treatments

LASIK

- A thin flap is created in the anterior cornea with a blade or laser
- The flap is reflected and the excimer laser is used to reshape the tissue beneath the flap
- The flap is then replaced and seals in place without sutures

PRK

- The epithelium is manually removed from the surface of the cornea
- The excimer laser is used to reshape the surface of the cornea
- The epithelium heals over the following 3 to 4 days

PIOL

- Surgically implanted device
- Natural lens remains intact
- Can treat high myopia

Refractive lens exchange

- Surgical removal of the natural lens
- Placement of intraocular lens
- Results in loss of accommodation
- Can treat high hyperopia or myopia

---

treatments are sometimes an option when the patient has adequate corneal thickness. If there is concern about corneal thickness, young patients with myopia are often better candidates for PIOL implantation.

Moderate-to-high Hyperopia

Because there is no PIOL approved by the Food and Drug Administration for the treatment of hyperopia, patients with hyperopia have more limited surgical options. Excimer laser treatments are most effective up to +4.00 D. The discrepancy between the limits for hyperopic and myopic treatment results from the relative ease in flattening the central cornea (myopic treatment) as contrasted with the difficulty in achieving a satisfactory optical result with steepening the central cornea (hyperopic treatment). Patients with hyperopia outside the range of excimer laser treatments have the option of a refractive lens exchange with IOL implantation.

Excimer lasers and PIOLs are not approved for use in the pediatric population. All of these treatments are available in the United States but are used on an off-label basis in children. A thorough discussion of the risks, benefits, and off-label nature of these treatments is necessary when planning for pediatric refractive surgery (**Box 3**).

CHALLENGES OF PEDIATRIC REFRACTIVE SURGERY

As in most aspects of medicine, children are not just small adults when considering refractive surgery. There are many unique challenges that arise when considering refractive surgery for the pediatric population. Paramount in the discussion of pediatric refractive surgery is the understanding of the fundamental difference between pediatric and adult indications for refractive surgery. Pediatric ophthalmologists must be

---

Box 3
Treatments for hyperopia

Low-to-moderate myopia and low hyperopia

- +3.00 to −8.00 D
- If adequate corneal thickness, absence of risk factors
- PRK or LASIK

High myopia

- PIOL
- Refractive lens exchange with or without IOL

Moderate-to-high hyperopia

- Refractive lens exchange

---

conscientious of safety concerns, but we cannot be so conservative that we prevent the pediatric population from benefiting from new technology. It has only been 30 to 35 years that pediatric ophthalmologists have routinely inserted an IOL after removing a cataract. Before this children with unilateral cataracts could only be corrected with a contact lens, and cases of bilateral cataracts were treated with very thick aphakic glasses or contact lenses. Visual rehabilitation was much less successful with such limited options, and contact lens complications in very young children are frequent. Through the work of forward-thinking pediatric ophthalmologists, children undergoing cataract surgery now have similar options as adults. Refractive surgery must be evaluated carefully as a potential option for a small segment of the pediatric population faced with specific vision problems.

Indications for Treatment

Adult refractive surgery is performed to eliminate the need for eyeglasses and contact lenses. It is an elective procedure that adults choose to reduce hassle with eyeglasses and contacts and simplify their lives. Pediatric refractive surgery is not ever an option simply to reduce the inconvenience of eyeglasses and contact lenses. It is only considered in cases where visual development or overall cognitive development is at risk because of the presence of an untreated refractive error. There are two primary conditions that are most commonly treated with pediatric refractive surgery: anisometropic amblyopia and bilateral high refractive error with neurodevelopmental disability.

Anisometropia occurs when the refractive error is very different between the two eyes. This can occur because of an underlying problem with one of the eyes (eg, glaucoma or myelinated nerve fiber layer) or can occur spontaneously. Depending on the degree of anisometropia, amblyopia may develop because of a poor retinal image from the eye with the higher refractive error. When this occurs, the first-line treatment is refractive correction with eyeglasses or contact lenses and then the use of an occlusive patch to treat the amblyopia. Most patients respond favorably to this treatment and the amblyopia reverses. When the vision is no longer at risk, the child wears eyeglasses or contact lenses until they become an adult. At this point they can choose to have elective refractive surgery. If the vision fails to respond to refractive correction and occlusive therapy, whether from poor compliance or primary failure to respond, then refractive surgery is considered.[12–15]

The other condition that has been addressed with pediatric refractive surgery is bilateral high refractive error with poor compliance with refractive correction.

Most infants are born hyperopic and shift toward emmetropia (no refractive error). Around the age of 7 to 9 years a certain percentage of children continue to shift and become myopic. There are genetic and environmental factors that are implicated in the progression of myopia. Myopia is mainly caused by axial growth of the eye. Currently, there is no way to predict which children will become myopic, how myopic they will be, and when the myopia will stop progressing. There are some general hereditary and environmental risk factors that are widely accepted. For example, children with at least one myopic parent are two to four times more likely to become myopic than a child whose parents are not myopic.[16] Myopia is much more prevalent in Chinese populations. This may be related to genetics and the prolonged school day and intensive reading to which Asian school age children are exposed. Animal experiments support the theory that prolonged reading can precipitate a myopic shift in populations at risk for myopia.[17] In a large prevalence study (refractive error study in children [RESC])[18,19] 55% of 15-year-old girls in rural China were myopic compared with 3% in Nepal.

Regardless of what causes severe myopia, there is no known prevention at this time; therefore, we must concentrate on refractive correction to help normal visual development. Most children with bilateral high refractive error take to wearing eyeglasses or contact lenses very rapidly and enjoy the clear vision provided by their correction. Most children who refuse their refractive correction have concurrent neurodevelopmental disorders including autism, brain injury, or genetic disorder. The stimulation of having eyeglasses on their face is often too bothersome to enjoy the benefits of clear vision. These children immediately remove their eyeglasses and in most cases do not allow the insertion of contact lenses. Children with mild refractive error, either hyperopic or myopic, can function well without correction and do not need refractive surgery. When the refractive error is greater than 3 to 4 D, then refractive surgery is considered.[20]

A secondary factor in this process is the timing of treatment. Visual development can occur up until the age of 7 to 9 years. Amblyopia that goes untreated past this point, and sometimes even younger, is very difficult if not impossible to reverse. Children with anisometropic amblyopia or bilateral high refractive errors should be identified; conservatively treated; and if treatment failure occurs, referred for surgery before reaching this age. Even after age 9, there is still the possibility for reversing a small amount of amblyopia, but effects are greater at a younger age (**Box 4**).

Box 4
Indications for pediatric refractive surgery

Anisometropic amblyopia

- High refractive error in only one eye with resultant amblyopia
- Failing conventional treatment with eyeglasses and patching
- Treatment at a younger age (<9 years) is preferred because of visual development

Bilateral high refractive error

- Unable/unwilling to wear refractive correction
- Often neurodevelopmentally disabled
- Younger treatment is preferred but can be performed at any age
- Postoperative cooperation may be a concern

Patient Cooperation

Adult laser and intraocular refractive surgeries are mostly outpatient procedures using only topical anesthesia. The patient is instructed to fixate on the operating light or laser target to center the treatment and assist in surgical manipulation. When dealing with a pediatric population the cooperation of the patient is much more variable. Adolescent subjects are often able to lay still and self-fixate,[21] but in surgery performed to prevent amblyopia the children are often much too young and require sedation. In the United States, studies have reported brief general anesthesia during excimer laser procedures.[22,23] Intraocular surgeries have been performed with general anesthesia in a similar manner to pediatric cataract surgeries.

Another challenge arises when considering the logistics for administering anesthesia during excimer laser treatments. Excimer lasers are cumbersome pieces of equipment and are for the most part immobile. They are usually located in outpatient surgery centers or in the office of refractive surgeons, far from the pediatric anesthesiology needed to perform sedation. Excimer laser technology is also costly with a laser price of $100,000 or more. For the most part this problem has been solved by bringing the laser into a pediatric hospital setting, which is a solution not available to every clinician.

A final challenge of patient cooperation with pediatric refractive surgery is the difficulty in examining patients and administering postoperative medications. Adult patients can be trusted not to rub or manipulate their eye in the healing stages postoperatively and can be examined at the slit-lamp. In children, it is strongly encouraged to keep the eye or eyes covered for the first 3 to 7 days after surgery to prevent any manipulation and decrease the risk for postoperative infection. The surgeon must become proficient in efficient examinations and slit-lamp examination may not be feasible. Finally, compliance with postoperative medications is more important in the pediatric population than in the adult population. Children have a greater risk of developing postoperative corneal haze without the use of topical steroids. If this haze develops, it may exacerbate the amblyopia and temporarily negate the effects of the laser treatment.

Desired Postoperative Correction

Planning for refractive surgery in the adult population consists of targeting a plano (no refractive error) or monovision refraction depending on the age or activities of the patient. Planning treatment and targeting a postoperative refraction are more challenging and complicated in the pediatric population. For the younger pediatric population undergoing surgery to prevent amblyopia, the desired postoperative refraction is plano. For older children the ideal postoperative refraction has not been established. Because most children can tolerate a mild degree of hyperopia, a mildly hyperopic target may be appropriate in children who continue to have a natural myopic progression with growth. Although population studies have examined the growth of the eye and changes in refraction, it cannot be calculated for an individual eye at this time.[24] The key to these calculations is to keep in mind that the refractive error of the child changes with age and the refractive surgeon must have future options available to handle future refractive needs. Options for future treatments include surface retreatment after PRK, PIOL exchange, piggyback IOL, contact lenses as the child matures, and future LASIK after previous IOL.

More Challenging Refractive Errors

As discussed, it was discovered that using an excimer laser to treat high refractive errors often led to inferior optical and safety outcomes. The problem arises with pediatric refractive surgery because the patients brought to the attention of refractive surgeons are often those with very severe refractive errors. Many of these errors fall outside of the range of treatments accepted for laser refractive procedures. With the larger refractive corrections it is necessary to look to alternative procedures, such as PIOLs and refractive lens exchange.

FUTURE ROLE OF REFRACTIVE TECHNOLOGY IN CHILDREN
Refractive Surgery in the Adolescent Population

A recent publication by Mathers and coworkers[25] postulated that refractive surgery was safer than contact lenses. Through comparison of studies estimating the risk of vision loss from contact lens wear compared with laser vision correction they conclude that laser surgery is safer than contact lens wear. Although this assertion has been widely disputed and debated, it raises concerns about the safety of long-term contact lens wear. There is growing concern about the safety of contact lens usage in the preteenage and adolescent populations. These children are more likely to take risks with the care, usage, and hygiene of their lenses and products. In the future, laser correction may be the default choice when the child stops growing and the prescription is stable for greater than 1 year.

Identifying and Treating Highly Anisometropic Eyes Earlier

One of the greatest hurdles to the early treatment of anisometropia and subsequent amblyopia is the problem of identifying these children at a young age. This condition is often not discovered until routine grade school vision screening when the child is nearing the age of visual maturation. When discovered and treated before visual maturation, anisometropia can be successfully treated with traditional forms of therapy including spectacles, contact lenses, and occlusion therapy.[26] Future movement in pediatric ophthalmology and pediatrics may be to find modalities of identifying anisometropic children at an earlier age. It is possible that as the techniques, technology, and experience with these surgical procedures expand, refractive surgery will be considered in certain cases at the time of diagnosis.

SUMMARY

The emerging field of pediatric refractive surgery is an interesting marriage of the rapidly progressing field of refractive surgery and the traditionally ultraconservative field of pediatric ophthalmology. The refractive side offers its advanced technologies and the pediatric group is charged with making conscientious and practical decisions regarding their use in children. In cases of anisometropic amblyopia and bilateral high myopia, surgeons have found clinical situations in which refractive surgery has been effective, safe, and beneficial.

Overall pediatric refractive surgery shows great promise in its ability to help a small segment of the pediatric population. Maximizing visual potential in patients who have often failed traditional therapies is the ultimate goal of these endeavors. Emerging techniques and technology may bring even more possibilities that could benefit an expanded population of infants, children, and adolescents.

REFERENCES

1. Trokel SL, Srinivasan R, Braren B. Excimer laser surgery of the cornea. Am J Ophthalmol 1983;96:710–5.
2. Kremer I, Kaplan A, Novikov I, et al. Patterns of late corneal scarring after photorefractive keratectomy in high and severe myopia. Ophthalmology 1999;106:467–73.

3. Moller-Pedersen T, Cavanagh HD, Petroll WM, et al. Stromal wound healing explains refractive instability and haze development after photorefractive keratectomy. Ophthalmology 2000;107:1235–45.
4. Marshall J, Trokel SL, Rothery S, et al. Long-term healing of the central cornea after photorefractive keratectomy using an excimer laser. Ophthalmology 1988; 95:1411–21.
5. Worst JG, van der Heijde G, Los LI. Refractive surgery for high myopia: the Worst-Fechner biconcave iris claw lens. Doc Ophthalmol 1990;75:335–41.
6. Zaldivar R, Davidorf JM, Oscherow S. Posterior chamber phakic intraocular lens for myopia of -8 to -19 diopters. J Refract Surg 1998;14:294–305.
7. Budo C, Hessloehl JC, Izak M, et al. Multicenter study of the Artisan phakic intraocular lens. J Cataract Refract Surg 2000;26:1163–71.
8. Menezo JL, Peris-Martinez C, Cisneros AL, et al. Phakic intraocular lenses to correct high myopia: Adatomed, Staar, and Artisan. J Cataract Refract Surg 2004;30:33–44.
9. Pop M, Payette Y. Initial results of endothelial cell counts after Artisan lens for phakic eyes: an evaluation of the United States Food and Drug Administration Ophtec Study. Ophthalmology 2004;111:309–17.
10. Stulting RD, John ME, Maloney RK, et al. Three-year results of Artisan/Verisyse phakic intraocular lens implantation results of the United States Food and Drug Administration clinical trial. Ophthalmology 2008;115(3):464–72.e1.
11. Lee KH, Lee JH. Long-term results of clear lens extraction for severe myopia. J Cataract Refract Surg 1996;22:1411–5.
12. Ali A, Packwood E, Lueder G, et al. Unilateral lens extraction for high anisometropic myopia in children and adolescents. J AAPOS 2007;11:153–8.
13. Alio JL, Artola A, Claramonte P, et al. Photorefractive keratectomy for pediatric myopic anisometropia. J Cataract Refract Surg 1998;24:327–30.
14. Assil KK, Sturm JM, Chang SH. Verisyse intraocular lens implantation in a child with anisometropic amblyopia: four-year follow-up. J Cataract Refract Surg 2007;33(11):1985–6.
15. Paysse EA, Coats DK, Hussein MA, et al. Long-term outcomes of photorefractive keratectomy for anisometropic amblyopia in children. Ophthalmology 2006;113: 169–76.
16. Mutti DO, Zadnik K. The utility of three predictors of childhood myopia: a Bayesian analysis. Vision Res 1995;35:1345–52.
17. Wallman J, McFadden S. Monkey eyes grow into focus. Nat Med 1995;1:737–9.
18. Zhao J, Pan X, Sui R, et al. Refractive error study in children: results from Shunyi District, China. Am J Ophthalmol 2000;129:427–35.
19. Pokharel GP, Negrel AD, Munoz SR, et al. Refractive error study in children: results from Mechi Zone, Nepal. Am J Ophthalmol 2000;129:436–44.
20. Tychsen L, Packwood E, Hoekel J, et al. Refractive surgery for uncorrected high bilateral myopia in children with neurobehavioral disorders: 1. Clear lens extraction and refractive lens exchange. J AAPOS 2006;10:357–63.
21. Phillips CB, Prager TC, McClellan G, et al. Laser in situ keratomileusis for treated anisometropic amblyopia in awake, autofixating pediatric and adolescent patients. J Cataract Refract Surg 2004;30:2522–8.
22. Mahfouz AK, Khalaf MA. Comparative study of 2 anesthesia techniques for pediatric refractive surgery. J Cataract Refract Surg 2005;31(12):2345–9.
23. Paysse EA, Hussein MA, Koch DD, et al. Successful implementation of a protocol for photorefractive keratectomy in children requiring anesthesia. J Cataract Refract Surg 2003;29:1744–7.

24. Hyman L, Gwiazda J, Hussein M, et al. Relationship of age, sex and ethnicity with myopia progression and axial elongation in the correction of myopia evaluation trial. Arch Ophthalmol 2005;123(7):977–87.
25. Mathers WD, Fraunfelder FW, Rich LF. Risk of Lasik surgery vs contact lenses. Arch Ophthalmol 2006;124(10):1510–1.
26. Kutschke PJ, Scott WE, Keech RV. Anisometropic amblyopia. Ophthalmology 1991;98:258–63.

The Lacrimal System

Faruk H. Örge, MD*, Charline S. Boente, MD, MS

KEYWORDS

- Lacrimal system • Epiphora (tearing) • Nasolacrimal duct obstruction
- Dacryocystocele • Tear duct probe

KEY POINTS

- Normal tear production may not be noticed until after a few weeks of life.
- Nasolacrimal duct obstruction (NLDO) is common in neonates (6% of all newborns).
- Most NLDOs spontaneously resolve with conservative management (70% by 6 months and 90% by 12 months of age).
- Surgical intervention for NLDO is in general straightforward and has a high success rate.
- Most pediatric ophthalmologists can perform a simple probing in the office if the infant is referred by 12 months of age. General anesthesia is required for children who fail a simple probing or who are referred at an older age (>12 months).

DEFINITION AND ANATOMY

1. The lacrimal system consists of the following structures (**Fig. 1**):
   a. The lacrimal gland is a bilobed exocrine gland arising from the epithelial cells of the superotemporal conjunctiva, located in the lacrimal gland fossa of the frontal bone. The 2 lobes, the lacrimal and the orbital lobes, contain ducts that secrete the aqueous portion of the tear film and are separated anatomically by the lateral horn of the levator aponeurosis, with the palpebral lobe located more distally. The palpebral lobe can often be visualized with eversion of the upper eyelid. Although the lacrimal gland receives both parasympathetic and sympathetic innervation, the secretion of tears is largely an action of parasympathetic innervation.[1]
   b. The accessory lacrimal glands of Krause and Wolfring are located within the conjunctival fornices and contribute approximately 10% of the tear secretion.
   c. The puncta are located on the upper and lower eyelids in the nasal corner at the junction of the pars ciliaris (lateral five-sixths containing lashes) and the pars lacrimalis (medial nonciliated one-sixth) and rest slightly inverted against the globe. The puncta serve as the exit point for tears from the conjunctival sac.[2]

Department of Ophthalmology and Visual Sciences, University Hospitals Rainbow Babies and Children's Hospital, Case Western Reserve University, Cleveland, OH, USA
* Corresponding author. 6001 B Landerhaven Drive, Mayfield Heights, OH 44124.
E-mail address: faruk.orge@uhhospitals.org

Pediatr Clin N Am 61 (2014) 529–539
http://dx.doi.org/10.1016/j.pcl.2014.03.002
0031-3955/14/$ – see front matter © 2014 Elsevier Inc. All rights reserved.

NLD Anatomy

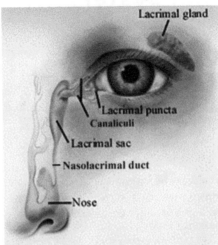

Fig. 1. Lacrimal system anatomy.

d. The ampulla extends vertically from each puncta about 2 mm.[2]
e. The canaliculi run medially about 90° from each ampulla approximately 8 mm and meet to form the common canaliculus, which opens into the lacrimal sac. Some individuals may have canaliculi that each open separately into the lacrimal sac. The valve of Rosenmuller, which is a mucosal flap separating the common canaliculus from the lacrimal sac, prevents tear reflux back into the canaliculi.[2]
f. The lacrimal sac runs vertically approximately 10 to 12 mm, with its superior portion extending above the common canaliculus. The lacrimal sac is lined with stratified columnar epithelium and lies in the lacrimal sac fossa.[2]
g. The nasolacrimal duct is also lined by stratified columnar epithelium and extends about 12 to 18 mm inferiorly and slightly laterally and posteriorly from the lacrimal sac. The duct empties into the inferior nasal meatus, with proper directional flow facilitated by the valve of Hasner, a mucosal flap separating the nasolacrimal duct from the nasal cavity.[2] The tears drain into the nose, and for this reason, your nose runs when you cry.
2. The tear film comprises the following layers:
a. The inner mucin layer allows for an even tear film layer over the ocular surface and is secreted by the goblet cells of the conjunctival epithelium.
b. The middle aqueous layer is secreted by the main and accessory lacrimal glands.
c. The outer oily layer maintains the tear film stability by preventing evaporation of the aqueous layer and is produced by the meibomian glands.[3] Without a healthy oily tear film, the tears evaporate, and this can lead to dry eye symptoms. The eye then tries to compensate by making more watery tears.

PHYSIOLOGY AND FUNCTION

Tear drainage is complex. The tears do not merely drain by gravitational flow. In a normal lacrimal pump system, blinking controlled by the orbicularis muscle causes closure of the canaliculi, with simultaneous opening of the lacrimal sac. The result is a negative pressure system, which draws tears into the sac via the ampullas and canaliculi. When the eyelids are opened, the puncta open, and a positive pressure in the lacrimal sac is reestablished, further pumping tears through the nasolacrimal duct to the nose.[3]

EMBRYOLOGY AND DEVELOPMENT

Development of the lacrimal gland begins around week 6 or 7 of gestation by linear thickening of epithelial cells originating from the conjunctival surface ectoderm between the nasal and maxillary processes. The lacrimal ducts are formed at about 3 months gestation, and canalization of the lacrimal drainage system continues from a cranial to caudal direction.[2,4] Although canalization of the nasolacrimal duct is typically complete at birth, full excretory function of the lacrimal glands does not occur until approximately 6 weeks after birth. Therefore, many newborns can be observed crying without tearing.[3,4] When parents are concerned because they do not see any tears, it is simple to reassure them that crying tears often does not occur for weeks.

CONGENITAL DISORDERS AND TREATMENT
Congenital Nasolacrimal Duct Obstruction

Clinical features
Nasolacrimal duct obstruction (NLDO) is the most common lacrimal system abnormality, occurring in up to 6% of all newborns.[5,6] The most common cause is incomplete canalization at the caudal end of the nasolacrimal duct, leaving an imperforate membrane at the valve of Hasner. Infants often present once tear production matures with chronic epiphora, eyelash matting, increased tear lake, or accumulation of mucoid discharge from the stasis of the tear lake and reflux of tears back into the lacrimal sac (**Fig. 2**). Diagnosis is often made by history and clinical examination alone. Although the clinical picture may look similar to conjunctivitis, patients do not have any discomfort or light sensitivity, and the bulbar conjunctiva (white of the eye) stays white and quiet. Chronic epiphora tends to cause the lashes to be singed down to the lower lid skin, and there may be skin changes, mainly in the lateral border of the lower lid because of the chronic irrigation and irritation in this region. There may be discomfort if the skin becomes red and chafed from chronic rubbing.

Digital massage over the lacrimal sac area resulting in reflux of fluid from the puncta, suggests a distal NLDO below the level of the sac.[2,5,6] A simple way to confirm the

NLDO

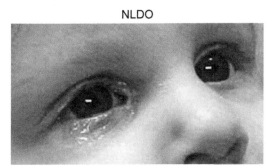

Fig. 2. NLDO of right side: patients do not have any discomfort or light sensitivity, and the bulbar conjunctiva (white of the eye) stays white and quiet. Chronic epiphora tends to cause the lashes to be singed down to the lower lid skin, and there may be skin changes, mainly in the lateral border of the lower lid, because of the chronic irrigation and irritation in this region.

diagnosis could be a dye disappearance test, in which fluorescein is applied to the inferior fornix using a fluorescein strip. The dye paints the existing tear film and is easily highlighted using cobalt blue light. In normal circumstances, the dye should disappear within 5 minutes via the normal irrigation system, but when the drainage system is blocked, it lingers or accumulates.

The differential diagnosis of NLDO should include conjunctivitis (eg, discharge, tearing, light sensitivity, foreign body sensation, redness), corneal abrasion (eg, pain, irritation, tearing, significant light sensitivity, history of trauma), and glaucoma (eg, tearing, light sensitivity, excessive blinking, cloudy cornea). Other causes include corneal or conjunctival foreign bodies, allergies, meningeal irritation, central nervous system tumors, abnormalities of the lids and lashes, or any other disorder of the cornea (congenital herpes) or conjunctiva causing irritation.

Recent studies indicate a higher incidence of associated ocular conditions that should be ruled out as well (eg, refractive error, anisometropia, amblyopia).[7] Therefore, a complete evaluation of the eyes by an ophthalmologist is crucial in cases of chronic tearing that presents at an unusual time, does not resolve as expected over time, or has any other associated findings such as conjunctival injection.

Management
Management of tearing and mattering associated with a tear duct obstruction is required, because this condition can cause not only social problems but also, although rare, serious infections in the lacrimal system, which may require more complex interventions such as dacryocystorhinostomy.

Nonsurgical External digital massage has been advocated as the primary method of conservative management. This technique consists of firmly massaging in a downward motion, starting from the area of the common canaliculus alongside the lacrimal sac and nasolacrimal duct. The increase in hydrostatic pressure within the lacrimal sac and duct is believed to rupture the membrane, resulting in a patent system.[2] Sometimes, topical antibiotics are needed to help control the mucus associated with bacterial overgrowth. Almost any antibiotic drop helps to control the mattering. Therefore, an inexpensive antibiotic should be started first. Parents should use the drops only for a short course (3–5 days), to prevent chemical irritation. Antibiotic drops can be used multiple times while waiting for resolution. Steroids should not be used. Before 10 months of age, conservative management with digital massage with or without topical antibiotics is recommended, because studies have consistently shown resolution by 6 months follow-up in 66% and 56% of unilateral and bilateral NLDO cases, respectively.[8]

Surgical Surgical approaches begin with probing and possible irrigation, which can be performed either in the office with topical anesthesia or in an operating room (OR) under general anesthesia. This technique typically starts with punctal dilation, followed by attempts to mechanically relieve the obstruction with irrigation. If irrigation fails, the surgeon proceeds with advancing a Bowman probe along the lacrimal drainage system (**Fig. 3**). Proficient knowledge of the anatomy is imperative, because proper technique is dependent on the surgeon's sense of touch when passing through structures. When an imperforate membrane is encountered, resistance and the associated obstruction are often relieved by gentle puncture of the probe. Improper passage of the probe may lead to the creation of a false passage, which can result in persistence of symptoms and potential scarring. If the child is asleep in the OR, accurate passage of the probe through the nasolacrimal system can be confirmed by introducing a second probe under the inferior nasal turbinate and detecting movement of the first probe.

NLD Probing

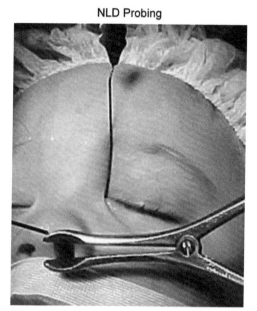

Fig. 3. Probing of left lacrimal drainage system.

If needed, direct inspection may be performed, with or without the aid of a nasal speculum, headlamp, or nasal endoscope.[9] A simple probing in the office takes only approximately 2 to 3 minutes, if the anatomy is normal.

Because of the data supporting resolution of NLDO in most cases with conservative management alone, many advocate deferred surgical treatment approaches. The timing of surgical management is controversial, but many suggest 12 months of age as the optimal time of surgical intervention, although it has been shown that the success rate of probing is 78% starting at 6 months of age to 36 months of age.[9,10]

Although highly dependent on the surgeon's level of comfort and the patient's ability to tolerate restraints, early in-office probing at 6 to 10 months of age has shown faster, more successful, and more cost-effective resolution of NLDO compared with observation until 12 months of age followed by probing under general anesthesia in a surgical facility. The argument against such an approach is that patients, most of whom would have otherwise resolved on their own, may undergo unnecessary probing, with possible negative psychological impacts.[11]

Some advocate the use of silicone tubing for intubation on initial probing as primary treatment. This procedure requires general anesthesia. Others advocate its use after 1 or more failed attempts of probing alone in the office. Other techniques used for persistent NLDOs after probing include repeat probing, balloon dilation, or rarely, deliberate fracture of the inferior turbinate to displace any bony obstruction to the nasolacrimal duct. Dacryocystorhinostomy, or the creation of a passage via a bony ostium between the lacrimal sac and nasal cavity, is typically reserved as a last resort when other options have failed.[9] For persistent NLDO, studies have shown success rates of 50%, 77%, and 84% for repeat probing, balloon dilation, and monocanalicular or bicanalicular tubing, respectively.[12,13] Because success is higher by placing a tube or dilating the system, this is usually suggested if the child is going to be under general anesthesia.

Congenital Dacryocystocele (Dacryocele)

Clinical features

A congenital dacryocystocele typically presents at or soon after birth as a bluish mass overlying the region of the lacrimal sac below the medial canthus (**Figs. 4** and **5**). Epiphora, inflammation, infection, corneal astigmatism, nasal cyst, or respiratory distress (in bilateral cases, because neonates are obligatory nasal breathers, and nasal cysts commonly accompany the dacryocystocele, obstructing the airway) may also be present. The outpouching represents the distention of the lacrimal sac and duct caused by an obstruction at both the valve of Hasner and the common canaliculus or valve of Rosenmuller. Most cases are unilateral.[14] It is important to rule out conditions such as encephalocele or meningocele, because these may appear as a bulge in the inner canthal area, but unlike the dacryocystocele, which is always located under the medial canthal tendon, these conditions are found to involve the area above the medial canthal tendon.

Management

Although dacryocystoceles are often resistant to resolution with digital massage, many begin treatment approaches conservatively with digital massage and/or topical antibiotics. Systemic antibiotics are needed if dacryocystitis is suspected. If conservative approaches fail to relieve the distention, and especially if dacryocystitis does not improve, probing with irrigation or marsupialization of the nasal cyst is recommended.[14]

Congenital Lacrimal Fistula

Clinical features

Although rare, congenital lacrimal fistulas are epithelial-lined tracts arising from the canaliculus, lacrimal sac, or nasolacrimal duct. The fistulas may exit to either the superior border of the upper eyelid tarsal plate or external at varying distances from the lateral or medial canthus (**Fig. 6**). Patients with a patent nasolacrimal duct are usually asymptomatic but may present with epiphora or purulent drainage from the fistula.[15] Associations have been made with Down syndrome, thalassemia, preauricular fistulae, hypospadias, and VACTERL (vertebral anomalies, anal atresia, cardiac malformation, tracheoesophageal fistula, renal abnormalities, and limb anomalies). Bilateral cases are rare but have been reported in association with Down syndrome.[16]

Management

If the patient is symptomatic and definitive treatment is desired, nasolacrimal duct probing and irrigation to relieve any obstruction, followed by excision of the fistula tract, are recommended.[15,16]

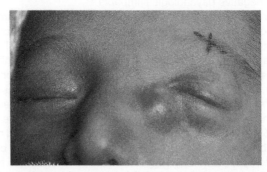

Fig. 4. Dacryocystocele: bluish, firm, nonmobile cyst seen below the medial canthal tendon.

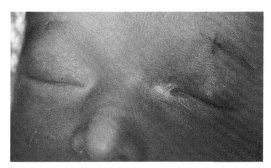

Fig. 5. Dacryocystocele: after decompression with tear duct probing.

Congenital Alacrima

Congenital alacrima (lack of tears) may present in association with abnormal conjunctival and eye development, such as in anophthalmos or cryptophthalmos. Alacrima may also present in association with triple A syndrome, a rare autosomal-recessive disease caused by a mutation of the AAAS gene, consisting of adrenal insufficiency, alacrima, and achalasia.[1,17]

Congenital Paradoxic Gustolacrimal Reflex (Crocodile Tears)

After damage to the facial nerve, lacrimation may occur with ipsilateral mastication. If this condition occurs congenitally, it is usually seen in association with ipsilateral Duane syndrome or lateral rectus palsy.[5]

Atresia of the Punctum or Canaliculus

Atresia of the punctum or canaliculus is rare. If the epithelium overlying the upper or lower punctum remains present, the outflow of tears is impeded and leads to epiphora, especially in cases of lower punctal atresia. Similarly, but even more rare, atresia of the canaliculus may occur. Management typically consists of probing or perforation, irrigation, and silicone tube placement.[5]

Lacrimal Gland Choristoma

Also rare, lacrimal gland choristoma consists of histologically normal lacrimal gland tissue found in abnormal locations, such as under the conjunctiva, at the limbus, within

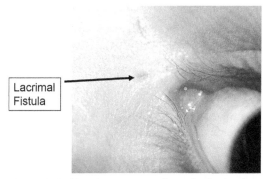

Lacrimal Fistula

Fig. 6. Lacrimal fistula: epithelial-lined tract arising from the lacrimal sac. Patient noticed to have tearing from this spot, but because there were no signs of infections, the patient was opted to be observed.

the sclera, or elsewhere in and around the eye. Simple excision is the treatment of choice, if needed.[5]

ACQUIRED DISORDERS AND TREATMENT
Dacryocystitis

Infection of the lacrimal sac occurs most commonly because of chronic tear retention and stasis from an NLDO. The presentation may be acute or chronic but consists of epiphora and erythematous distention or swelling below the medial canthal area, with or without pain. The most common pathogens are *Streptococcus* and *Staphylococcus* species. Treatment typically consists of warm compresses with oral antibiotics, or parenteral antibiotics in severe cases. Topical antibiotics are usually ineffective, and probing and irrigation should be avoided with active infection. If an abscess formation is suspected, incision and drainage may be required, although this carries an increased risk of lacrimal sac fistula formation. In cases of total NLDO or in chronic dacryocystitis, a dacryocystorhinostomy is often required.[2,3]

Dacryoadenitis

Rarely, noninfectious or, less commonly, infectious inflammation of the lacrimal gland may develop. Noninfectious dacryoadenitis can occur as a result of a malignancy. Rarely, the lacrimal gland may become infected from direct extension from an adjacent source, from trauma, or hematogenously, such as from tuberculosis or Epstein-Barr virus.[3]

Canaliculitis

Infection of the canaliculus can be caused by a variety of bacterial, viral, or mycotic organisms, but the most common cause is *Actinomyces israelii*, a filamentous gram-positive rod. Canaliculitis presents with unilateral epiphora, in addition to a mucopurulent conjunctivitis, a dilated pouting punctum, swelling of the canaliculus, and expression or mucopurulent discharge. Infection by *Actinomyces* often results in the formation of concretions or canalicular stones, shown on expression or with canaliculotomy. In contrast to dacryocystitis, lacrimal sac distention or inflammation is absent. In isolated canaliculitis, treatment consists of a stepwise approach, beginning with warm compresses, digital massage, and topical antibiotics, with or without oral antibiotics. If stones are present, punctal curettage may be attempted, but removal may require a canaliculotomy of the horizontal canaliculus from a conjunctival approach.[2,3]

Punctal or Canalicular Stenosis

In children, acquired canalicular stenosis can result from viral infections, such as varicella, which produce inflammation, leading to subepithelial fibrosis and scarring. Other causes of acquired punctal or canalicular stenosis include medications, trauma, neoplasms, and bacterial or mycotic infections.[1]

Association with Facial Abnormalities

Craniofacial anomalies may affect normal function and development of the lacrimal system, predisposing the patient to the conditions mentioned earlier.

CLINICAL ASSESSMENT
History and External Examination

In the case of epiphora, thorough and goal-directed history and physical examination are essential. The duration, frequency, unilaterality, and appearance of the tearing should be questioned. A systematic examination should be performed, including examination of the medial canthal region for any distention or discoloration, eyelid margin for evaluation of puncta patency, location of epiphora or discharge, and any identifiable sources of increased reflex tearing. Attention to signs of possible infectious conjunctivitis or dacryocystitis, blepharitis, trichiasis, or epiblepharon is important for determining the cause of tearing and mattering.[3]

Testing

Pediatricians' and ophthalmologists' tests
Dye disappearance test The dye disappearance test is commonly used in the evaluation of NLDO in children. Similar to the tear breakup time (TBUT) test, fluorescein is placed in the inferior fornix of both eyes and then observed under a cobalt blue light. Attention is drawn to the tear film, and the amount of dye remaining after 5 minutes is noted, accounting for any asymmetry between eyes. In a normal lacrimal system, the tear film should be clear after 5 minutes.[18]

Lacrimal sac compression Using pressure over the lacrimal sac fossa with an index finger or cotton-tipped applicator stick, any mucous or mucopurulent material expressed with upward motion toward the canaliculus and puncta indicates an obstruction, most commonly in the nasolacrimal duct.[18]

Ophthalmologists' tests
Tear breakup time (TBUT) To evaluate the TBUT, fluorescein is placed in the inferior fornix of both eyes, the patient blinks, and the time to disruption of the tear film on the cornea is measured via observation under a cobalt blue light, typically with a slit lamp. A TBUT of less than 10 seconds is suggestive of tear film instability caused by inadequate tear composition.[18]

Schirmer I and Schirmer II test The Schirmer I and Schirmer II tests are performed without and with anesthetic eyedrops, respectively. The test consists of measuring the extent of tear wetting on standardized strips. The lower eyelid margin is dried, and a sterile filter paper strip is folded and placed overhanging the outer one-third of each lower eyelid margin, making sure not to contact the cornea. After 5 minutes, the strips are removed, and the extent of wetting is measured along the millimeter scale of the strips. A measurement of 10 or less is suggestive of moderate dry eye syndrome, and 5 or less suggests severe dry eye syndrome.[18,19]

Jones I and Jones II test The Jones I test evaluates physiologic conditions by instilling fluorescein in the conjunctival sac, followed by placing a cotton-tipped applicator under the inferior turbinate to retrieve dye at 2 and 5 minutes. Positive dye recovery indicates a patent and functional nasolacrimal drainage system, although recovery times may be variable, and false-negative results are frequent. A negative Jones I test does not differentiate between inadequate physiologic function and anatomic obstruction. If the Jones I test is negative, the Jones II test can be performed to confirm anatomic patency. The conjunctival sac is cleared of remaining dye, and clear saline is irrigated through the nasolacrimal system. Retrieval from the nose suggests normal anatomy, whereas reflux containing fluorescein suggests an obstruction. Because of the high false-positive and false-negative rates as well as the technical difficulty of performing these tests, the Jones I and Jones II tests are infrequently used.[20]

Irrigation Irrigation of the nasolacrimal system is often considered the gold standard for evaluation of anatomic obstruction. The puncta are dilated, and saline is injected using a lacrimal cannula. If saline refluxes through the same punctum being injected, an obstruction at the level of the canaliculus is present. If saline refluxes through the opposite punctum, an obstruction distal to the common canaliculus is present. Passage of saline through the nose indicates an anatomically patent system, and a mixed result suggests a partial obstruction or narrowing.[20]

Dacryocystogram A dacryocystogram may be obtained if the cause of the nasolacrimal abnormality is unclear. This test begins with intubation, then irrigation of the nasolacrimal system with a radiopaque substance, followed by a series of images captured, most often using a digital subtraction technique. Both sides are tested and compared for narrowing, distention, fistulae, blocking, or other anatomic anomalies.[20]

Nasal endoscopy Nasal endoscopy can be performed to obtain direct visualization to evaluate nasal anatomy, such as before or during surgery.

Computed tomography and magnetic resonance imaging Although not typically used as first-line evaluation for a patient with epiphora or dry eye syndrome, computed tomography can be used most often in suspected bony abnormalities, such as in trauma or craniofacial deformities. Magnetic resonance imaging is typically used in suspected soft tissue abnormalities, such as malignancy.[20]

REFERENCES

1. Ellis FD. Lacrimal system. In: Wright KW, Spiegel PH, editors. Pediatric ophthalmology and strabismus. 2nd edition. New York: Springer; 2003. p. 313–20.
2. Kanski JJ, Bowling B. Lacrimal drainage system. In: Clinical ophthalmology: a systematic approach. 7th edition. Edinburgh (United Kingdom): Elsevier; 2011. p. 65–78.
3. Holds JB, Chang WJ, Durairaj VD, et al. Development, anatomy, and physiology of the lacrimal secretory and drainage systems and abnormalities of the lacrimal secretory and drainage systems. In: Skuta GL, Cantor LB, Weiss JS, editors. Basic and clinical science course (BCSC) section 7: orbit, eyelids, and lacrimal system. San Francisco (CA): American Academy of Ophthalmology (AAO); 2012. p. 243–78.
4. Chalam KV, Ambati BK, Beaver HA, et al. Ocular development. In: Skuta GL, Cantor LB, Weiss JS, editors. Basic and clinical science course (BCSC) section 2: fundamentals and principles of ophthalmology. San Francisco (CA): American Academy of Ophthalmology (AAO); 2012. p. 140.
5. Calhoun JH. Disorders of the lacrimal apparatus in infancy and childhood. In: Nelson LB, Calhoun JH, Harley RD, editors. Pediatric ophthalmology. 3rd edition. Philadelphia: WB Saunders; 1991. p. 325–33.
6. Christian CJ, Nelson LB. Lacrimal system disorders in infants and children. Ophthalmol Clin North Am 1990;3(2):239–47.
7. Piotrowski JT, Diehl NN, Mohney BG. Neonatal dacryostenosis as a risk factor for anisometropia. Arch Ophthalmol 2010;128(9):1166–9.
8. Pediatric Eye Disease Investigator Group. Resolution of congenital nasolacrimal duct obstruction with nonsurgical management. Arch Ophthalmol 2012;130(6):730–4.
9. Raab EL, Aaby AA, Bloom JN, et al. The lacrimal drainage system. In: Skuta GL, Cantor LB, Weiss JS, editors. Basic and clinical science course (BCSC) section 6: pediatric ophthalmology and strabismus. San Francisco (CA): American Academy of Ophthalmology (AAO); 2012. p. 203–10.
10. Pediatric Eye Disease Investigator Group. Primary treatment of nasolacrimal duct obstruction with probing in children less than four years old. Ophthalmology 2008;115(3):577–84.

11. Pediatric Eye Disease Investigator Group. A randomized trial comparing the cost-effectiveness of 2 approaches for treating unilateral nasolacrimal duct obstruction. Arch Ophthalmol 2012;130(12):1525–33.
12. Pediatric Eye Disease Investigator Group. Repeat probing for treatment of persistent nasolacrimal duct obstruction. J AAPOS 2009;13(3):306–7.
13. Pediatric Eye Disease Investigator Group. Balloon catheter dilation and nasolacrimal intubation for treatment of nasolacrimal duct obstruction following a failed probing. Arch Ophthalmol 2009;127(5):633–9.
14. Shekunov J, Griepentrog GJ, Diehl NN, et al. Prevalence and clinical characteristics of congenital dacryocystocele. J AAPOS 2010;14(5):417–20.
15. Blanksma LJ, vd Pol BA. Congenital fistulae of the lacrimal gland. Br J Ophthalmol 1980;64:515–7.
16. Singh M, Sing U. Bilateral congenital lacrimal fistula in Down syndrome. Middle East Afr J Ophthalmol 2013;20(3):263–4.
17. Dixit A, Chow G, Sarkar A. Neurologic presentation of triple A syndrome. Pediatr Neurol 2011;45(5):347–9.
18. Wilson FM, Blomquist PH. External examination and anterior segment exam. In: Skuta GL, Cantor LB, Weiss JS, editors. Practical ophthalmology: a manual for beginning residents. 6th edition. San Francisco (CA): American Academy of Ophthalmology (AAO); 2009. p. 127–54, 188, 210.
19. The definition and classification of dry eye disease: report of the definition and classification subcommittee of the International Dry Eye Workshop. Ocul Surf 2007;5(2):75–92.
20. Dutton JJ, White JJ. Imaging and clinic evaluation of the lacrimal drainage system. In: Cohen AJ, Mercandetti M, Brazzo BG, editors. The lacrimal system: diagnosis, management, and surgery. New York: Springer; 2006. p. 74–98.

Periocular Hemangiomas and Lymphangiomas

Rachel E. Reem, MD[a],*, Richard P. Golden, MD[b]

KEYWORDS

- Periocular hemangioma • Orbital lymphatic malformation
- Venous-lymphatic malformation • Percutaneous sclerotherapy • Amblyopia

KEY POINTS

- Hemangiomas are the most common benign tumor of childhood.
- Most hemangiomas do not require treatment, but periocular hemangiomas should be followed closely.
- Ocular sequelae of unchecked vascular malformation growth can include amblyopia, strabismus, proptosis, corneal exposure, or optic nerve injury/atrophy.
- Recent shifts in hemangioma treatment paradigm have occurred: from systemic and intralesional steroids to systemic propranolol and topical timolol.
- Amblyogenic vascular anomalies (those involving the eyelids, those affecting eyelid closure, or those with suspected proptosis) should prompt referral to ophthalmology.

INTRODUCTION

Pediatric vascular anomalies include a diverse spectrum of tumors and malformations that can be found anywhere on the body, but elicit a unique set of sequelae when found near the eye. The most common of these are capillary hemangiomas,[1–5] followed closely in incidence by cavernous hemangiomas.[3] Additional vascular anomalies that are less frequent, but no less clinically significant, include arteriovenous malformations, lymphangiomas, angiosarcomas, and hemangiopericytomas.

Each of the above listed lesions, when found near the eye, has the potential to affect ocular health and vision. Potential sequelae include amblyopia (deprivational or refractive), strabismus, ocular motility restriction, globe proptosis, corneal exposure, and optic nerve injury/atrophy. Consequently, it is crucial for pediatricians to be familiar with these lesions, their potential ocular sequelae, and clinical signs which should precipitate referral to an ophthalmologist.

[a] Department of Ophthalmology, Nationwide Children's Hospital, 700 Children's Drive ED5 F2, Columbus, OH 43205, USA; [b] Department of Ophthalmology, Nationwide Children's Hospital, 555 South 18th Street, Suite 4C, Columbus, OH 43205, USA
* Corresponding author.
E-mail address: rachel.reem@nationwidechildrens.org

Pediatr Clin N Am 61 (2014) 541–553
http://dx.doi.org/10.1016/j.pcl.2014.03.007
0031-3955/14/$ – see front matter © 2014 Elsevier Inc. All rights reserved.

HEMANGIOMA
Extent of Problem

Infantile hemangiomas are the most common benign tumor of childhood, being found in anywhere from 2.6% to 10% of the pediatric population up to 1 year of age.[1,2,6,7] They can be found on any part of the body, but 38% to 60% are found in the head and neck.[1,8] Although one-third of these lesions are present at birth, most develop over the first year of life and progress through proliferative and involutional phases. Typically, hemangiomas reach 80% of their final size by the time a child is 5 months old.[9]

Superficial lesions can present with a bright red, lobulated, placoid appearance (hence the term "strawberry nevus"), or deeper lesions can present as a more bluish-purple, subcutaneous mass. Hemangiomas involving the orbit may present with displacement of the globe, proptosis (axial displacement of the globe), or ocular motility limitations. Lesions can sometimes display both superficial and deep components (**Fig. 1**). They are usually solitary, but up to 20% of affected infants have multiple lesions. Hemangiomas can also be found in either a localized or a segmental (territorial) distribution.[4–6,9–11] They tend to grow more in depth than radially or territorially.[9]

Hemangiomas generally proceed through 3 phases of growth. The initial proliferative phase is characterized by a period of rapid growth, usually in the first 3 to 6 months. This period of rapid growth is followed by a period of quiescence and then by involution. The involutional phase typically begins in the lesion's center and progresses throughout the first decade of life, mostly occurring by age 5.[7,9,10,12]

A small subset of hemangiomas presents at birth. These congenital hemangiomas often display marked growth during the proliferative phase and tend to involute much faster than those lesions that present in the weeks to months after birth.[13]

It is worth noting that there is some question as to whether the quiescent period is truly a distinct phase. Recent advances in understanding of the molecular basis of hemangioma growth and involution suggest that the proliferative and involution phases are mediated, in effect, by a "balance of power" between growth factors and factors driving apoptosis. It would stand to reason, then, that an apparent quiescent phase could simply be the junction between proliferative and involutional phases, and not itself a distinct phase.[9]

Mulliken and Glowacki[14] classified common pediatric vascular lesions on the basis of endothelial cell characteristics. They found that during the proliferative phase, hemangiomas were found to have endothelial cell hyperplasia with and without lumina, as

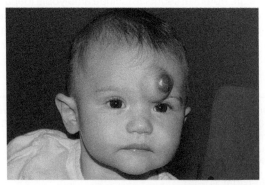

Fig. 1. Mixed hemangioma. Brow hemangioma displaying both superficial and deep components.

well as thickening of the underlying basement membrane. During the involution phase, fibrosis and fat deposition dominate the histologic appearance of hemangiomas. In contrast, those lesions characterized as vascular malformations demonstrate large vascular channels with a unilamellar basement membrane lined by flat endothelium, without proliferation of endothelial cells.

Cause, Contributory Factors, Risk Factors

Infantile hemangiomas are vascular tumors composed of clusters of endothelial cells with increased mitosis surrounding small vascular spaces. Angiogenesis-related cellular markers (type IV collagenase, basic fibroblastic growth factor, vascular endothelial growth factor, urokinase, and E-selectin) have been identified in proliferative phase hemangiomas.[15] As they involute, there is a progressive decrease in the cellular component of endothelial and mast cells, and the lesion becomes mostly composed of fibrous and fatty tissue. Finally, the vascular components atrophy completely.[7]

Patients with infantile hemangioma are more likely to be female gender(by a ratio of 2 or 3 to 1),[7,16] fair-skinned, premature, or a product of multiple gestation. Advanced maternal age, placenta previa, and pre-eclampsia also seem to be influencing factors, but this may be confounded by the fact that these prenatal risk factors are simultaneous risk factors for premature birth.[5] There is no known inheritance pattern, and siblings of children with infantile hemangiomas do not seem to have higher risk for developing the lesions than does the general population.[1]

Mast cells appear to play a pathophysiologic role in the proliferative phase of infantile hemangiomas. Glowacki and Mulliken[17] demonstrated that mast cells were present in proliferative phase hemangiomas in concentrations more than 5-fold greater than normal skin and 10-fold greater than in involuting hemangiomas. In vitro studies have also suggested that estrogen and hypoxia synergistically stimulate endothelial cell proliferation.[18]

Sequelae of the problem

Although most infantile hemangiomas, once involuted, display little sign of their earlier presence, some can become problematic, primarily because of location. If located in the airway or the mouth, these lesions can interfere with breathing or feeding. Visceral hemangiomas can create life-threatening sequelae by virtue of the fact that lesions with a high flow pattern can precipitate high-output cardiac failure and anemia. When lesions are found in the periocular region, several complications can occur.[4,5,8,12]

Amblyopia is a condition whereby the vision of the affected eye is reduced because of refractive error, strabismus, or occlusion. It is one of the most common sequelae of periocular hemangiomas, occurring in 43% to 60% of affected patients.[19,20] Amblyopia can occur as a result of obstruction of the visual axis, which is especially common for hemangiomas involving the eyelids (**Fig. 2**). In addition, the lesion can exert pressure on the eye itself, creating a change in refractive error and often inducing astigmatism. Astigmatism alone can cause amblyopia of the affected eye if severe enough.

Deeper hemangiomas involving the orbit can create proptosis. If severe, this can hamper eyelid closure and cause exposure keratopathy, a potentially vision-threatening deterioration of the cornea. In addition, if the optic nerve is stretched or compressed by the lesion, injury and subsequent optic atrophy with vision loss can occur. Ocular motility may be affected as well, which can lead to strabismus and possible strabismic amblyopia.[7] Ulceration is the most common complication of infantile hemangiomas and can occur on periocular lesions as well as those located elsewhere.[21]

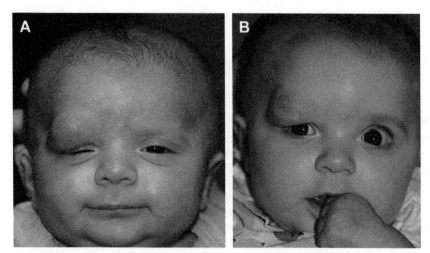

Fig. 2. Ocular sequelae of periocular hemangiomas, large brow hemangioma causing deprivational amblyopia. (*A*) 7-week-old infant presenting with large brow hemangioma obstructing the visual axis, on systemic propranolol therapy. (*B*) Same infant at 4 months, after systemic propranolol, topical timolol, and intralesional steroid ×2. Note improvement in eyelid opening, but pupillary light reflex suggests strabismus, brought on by deprivational amblyopia in the earlier weeks of the lesion's course.

Clinical Assessment

Most infantile hemangiomas can be diagnosed purely based on their characteristic appearance. Superficial hemangiomas appear as bright red, lobulated lesions, as their name "strawberry hemangioma" describes. Deeper hemangiomas present as bluish-purple-hued masses. Orbital hemangiomas may display few signs aside from proptosis of the globe, but their differential diagnosis includes other mass lesions, such as rhabdomyosarcoma, neuroblastoma, and lymphatic malformations. Thus, it is crucial to arrive at a correct diagnosis quickly.

In general, lesions at greater risk for complications include airway-threatening or sight-threatening lesions, lesions with a segmental distribution, larger lesion size, and facial location.[5] Location of the lesion is a key factor in determining whether to refer a patient to an ophthalmologist or other subspecialist, and whether to obtain imaging tests. Lesions located on the eyelids or in the orbit, causing proptosis, can potentially threaten vision. These lesions should be monitored very closely by an ophthalmologist. Patients demonstrating more than 5 cutaneous hemangiomas anywhere on the body should be considered for imaging to evaluate for visceral hemangiomas.[8,22] Any patient with proptosis of the eye should have imaging performed.

The optimal imaging study for hemangiomas is magnetic resonance imaging (MRI). The characteristic morphology and architecture are captured particularly well by high-resolution thin-section T2-weighted images with fat suppression, or T1-weighted images with gadolinium. The former modality highlights the internal lobular structure of the hemangioma. The latter modality displays hemangiomas at a signal intensity equal to or slightly higher than that of muscle, with signal voids within and around the periphery of the lesion. Gadolinium injection displays marked contrast enhancement. Rhabdomyosarcoma lesions, if highly vascularized, can mimic hemangioma characteristics on MRI.

Computed tomographic (CT) scanning demonstrates hemangiomas as lobulated enhancing masses with irregular margins, but does not demonstrate internal structure as well as does MRI. Ultrasonography is a cost-effective modality that does display characteristic variable internal reflectivity, and its highest value lies in monitoring lesions for changes over the course of time.[7,10]

Kasabach-Merritt Syndrome

Initially described in 1940, Kasabach-Merritt syndrome is characterized by consumptive coagulopathy, with resulting thrombocytopenia, in the context of hemangiomata.[23] Occasionally, the hemangiomas can be occult, but rapidly enlarging cutaneous hemangiomas can also be related to this syndrome. Patients demonstrate severe thrombocytopenia and usually have some degree of microangiopathic hemolysis. MRI findings in Kasabach-Merritt syndrome are similar to those of typical hemangiomas, but hemosiderin deposits can help identify sites of red cell destruction. Angiography can sometimes be useful for determining the extent of vasculature before embolization therapy. Management of this syndrome includes supportive treatment, surgical or compression therapy, vascular embolization, and in rare cases, radiotherapy, corticosteroids, interferon-α, and chemotherapy.[24]

PHACE Syndrome

Large segmental facial or scalp hemangiomas should prompt consideration of other congenital anomalies, such as in the PHACE syndrome. This syndrome's acronym name refers to posterior fossa abnormalities, hemangioma, arterial lesions, cardiac abnormalities (including aortic coarctation), and eye abnormalities. Major diagnostic criteria for this syndrome include anomalies of the major cerebral arteries, posterior fossa anomalies such as Dandy-Walker complex or cerebellar hypoplasia/dysplasia, aortic arch anomalies, sternal defects, and ocular abnormalities of the posterior segment. Minor criteria include persistent cerebral embryonic arteries (other than the trigeminal artery), extra-axial brain lesion with features consistent with hemangioma, ventricular septal defect, hypopituitarism or ectopic thyroid, and ocular abnormalities of the anterior segment. In patients with lesions that elicit suspicion for PHACE syndrome, brain imaging, echocardiogram, and formal ophthalmologic evaluation should be performed.[25,26]

Management

There have been several major paradigm shifts in the management of hemangiomas. In the 1940s and 1950s, irradiation was a common intervention (although some decried such aggressive treatment in lesions that are typically self-limited).[4,20,23] Radiotherapy can still be effective in select cases, although it should be reserved for those situations in which there are no viable alternatives.[7]

In the 1960s, corticosteroid therapy was the mainstay of treatment of problematic hemangiomas.[27] Multiple subsequent reports in the literature have indicated regression of hemangiomas in response to systemic administration of corticosteroids.[7,28–30] The most commonly recommended oral corticosteroid is prednisone, dosed at either 1 to 2 mg/kg daily or 2 to 4 mg/kg every other day.[1,7] Mechanisms by which corticosteroids induce hemangioma regression are not well understood. Systemic complications are a potential pitfall, and clinicians must be on the lookout for adrenal suppression, growth delay, gastrointestinal upset, hypertension, and increased susceptibility to infection.[4,7,27–29]

Intralesional steroid injection has also been an option for hemangioma treatment. Local administration of corticosteroids further decreases the risks of systemic complications, although reports of central retinal artery occlusion (a condition that causes severe vision loss) can be found in the literature.[31,32] In addition, localized atrophy (of fat and subcutaneous tissues), hypopigmentation, subcutaneous deposits of corticosteroid material, and local eyelid necrosis have all been reported.[1,7,31,32] Nevertheless, the overall complication rate is considered to be low. Injections may need to be repeated more than once, typically at intervals as often as every 4 to 6 weeks. Vaccinations with live-attenuated virus should be avoided for 4 weeks before or after intralesional steroid injection.

Surgical excision remains an option for lesions unresponsive to medical management. However, the logistics of surgery can be problematic because of the unencapsulated nature of these lesions and the potential for uncontrolled bleeding. Although surgery is a less attractive option than medical management, it is certainly a viable one for refractory lesions.[7,33–35]

Other less common treatment options have included cryotherapy, interferon-α, bleomycin, vincristine, embolization, and laser therapy.[1,4,7] These treatments have generally been reserved for lesions refractory to more common treatments.

The currently preferred treatment modality was discovered serendipitously by Léauté-Labrèze and colleagues[36] and reported in 2008. Two infants with hemangiomas developed cardiac issues and were subsequently placed on systemic propranolol. Their hemangiomas regressed within the first week of systemic β-blocker initiation. In light of this, 9 other infants with severe or disfiguring hemangiomas were also placed on systemic propranolol, achieving similar results. Initial changes in the lesions including softening and diminished intensity in color were seen within the first 24 hours of therapy. This discovery sparked the most recent paradigm shift in hemangioma management, culminating in a consensus statement on systemic propranolol for hemangiomas in 2013.[37] Indeed, β-blockers now seem to have replaced corticosteroids as the first-line therapy for problematic infantile hemangiomas.[37,38] Hypotension is the most commonly reported serious complication thus far. Other potentially serious complications include bradycardia, hypoglycemia or hypoglycemic seizure, hyperkalemia, and bronchial hyperreactivity. Less serious complications commonly reported include sleep disturbances, somnolence, gastrointestinal upset, and cold/mottled extremities.

Current recommendations for systemic propranolol were made in a consensus statement in 2013. Although the authors stress that evidence-based recommendations are not yet available, a comprehensive review of the literature to date was performed, and conservative recommendations based on that large body of work were made.

Pretreatment considerations

Contraindications to propranolol therapy include cardiogenic shock, sinus bradycardia, hypotension, greater than first-degree heart block, heart failure, bronchial asthma, and hypersensitivity to propranolol. Pretreatment assessment should include a careful history, evaluating for key elements of these conditions, and a careful examination including cardiac and pulmonary systems. Electrocardiogram screening is recommended for patients in whom the heart rate is less than normal for age, patients with a history of arrhythmia, and patients with a family history of congenital cardiac issues, arrhythmias, or connective tissue disorders. Infants with PHACE syndrome theoretically have an increased risk of stroke with propranolol therapy. However, these infants often are at high risk for medical morbidities and permanent facial scarring, and as such, can also be prime candidates for propranolol therapy. There are some cautiously positive reports of successful propranolol therapy in PHACE syndrome,[26,37] but these patients should be evaluated carefully for induction, using head and neck MRI/magnetic resonance angiography as well as cardiac imaging with special attention to the aortic arch. Comanagement with neurology may be indicated if a patient with PHACE syndrome would be at higher risk of stroke while on systemic propranolol.[26,37]

Induction of systemic propranolol The consensus recommendation for target dose of propranolol is 1 to 3 mg/kg/d divided into 3 times daily dosing with a minimum of 6 hours between doses. The median dose reported in the literature is 2 mg/kg/d. The final dose should be titrated up from a low starting point, with special attention paid to dose response. Initiation in an inpatient setting is recommended for infants of a corrected gestational age of 8 weeks or less, as well as those with comorbidities such as those described above, regardless of age.

Monitoring

Baseline heart rate and blood pressure should be measured before initiation, and these measurements should be repeated at 1 and 2 hours after administration of the first dose (peak effect of propranolol being achieved 1–3 hours after administration). Dose response is most drastic after the first dose, so there is no further need to monitor vital signs after subsequent doses in patients more than 8 weeks of age with no comorbidities. A set of measurements should be repeated after the target dose is achieved. Holter monitoring is not thought to be routinely necessary at this time. Serum glucose measurements are not recommended as part of routine monitoring, but parents should be educated on regular feeding and avoidance of prolonged fasting. Propranolol should be discontinued during illness, especially if the child is not inclined to eat. Care should be taken in patients undergoing sedation for procedures or imaging studies as well.

Hypotension is the most commonly reported serious complication thus far. Other potentially serious complications include bradycardia, hypoglycemia or hypoglycemic seizure, hyperkalemia, and bronchial hyperreactivity. Less serious complications commonly reported included sleep disturbances, somnolence, gastrointestinal upset, and cold/mottled extremities.

In addition to systemic β-blocker therapy, topical timolol has also been found efficacious in the treatment of superficial hemangiomas (**Fig. 3**). Typically, 0.5% timolol maleate drops, or 0.25% timolol maleate gel,[39] is applied to lesions 2 to 3 times daily. This therapy was first described by Guo and Ni in 2010,[39] and subsequent literature supports the finding that it is effective for more superficial lesions, even in cases of infants with PHACE syndrome.[40–44] Further work is needed to provide stronger evidence-based support for this therapy, but it seems to have similarly promising prospects to those of systemic propranolol.

In light of all treatment options available, one must not forget to address parental reactions and fears in response to their children's condition. Reports suggest that emotional reactions of parents were similar to those of parents whose children had permanent malformations. Parents have reported unsolicited comments from strangers, including abuse accusations, and may experience general frustration with medical care, particularly in cases whereby no active intervention is being pursued.[4,45] Showing parents before and after photographs, in addition to documenting hemangiomas with photography at each visit for comparison, may help parents in coping with their child's diagnosis.[45,46] In addition, although most hemangiomas achieve 80% of their final size by age 5 months, this is also the most common age for referral to dermatologists. Earlier referral may help in the assessment and optimal treatment of these

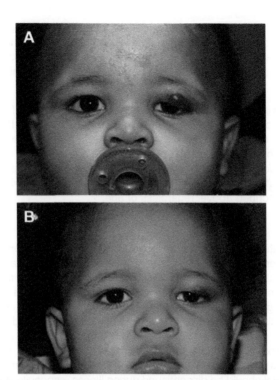

Fig. 3. Topical timolol for superficial hemangioma. (*A*) An 8-month-old infant at initial presentation with superficial upper eyelid hemangioma. (*B*) Same patient after 6 months of topical timolol administered twice daily. Systemic propranolol was started soon after this picture for the residual deep components of the hemangioma.

lesions.[9] Earlier referral for hemangiomas that are likely to be problematic may also help allay parental concerns.

LYMPHANGIOMA (LYMPHATIC AND VENOUS-LYMPHATIC MALFORMATIONS)
Extent of Problem

Lymphangiomas are a common orbital space-occupying lesion. They are benign hamartomatous vascular tumors that differ from hemangiomas in that they do not display proliferating endothelial cells. They account for 25% of orbital vasculogenic lesions,[47] and 1% to 3% of all orbital masses.[48] Like hemangiomas, they can present in both the superficial and the deep orbital space. They consist of dilated, thin-walled vascular chambers lined with endothelium and supported by fibrous stroma and contain a proteinaceous material reminiscent of lymph.[7,49] They can be classified as microcystic, macrocystic, or mixed.[47,50]

There is some controversy as to the nomenclature of lymphangiomas. The term "lymphangioma" does not accurately describe their histologic characteristics, which can include blood or blood products, and both vascular and lymphatic structures.[51–53] Furthermore, some think that the suffix "oma" connotes neoplastic or replicating cells, which these lesions do not have.[14] They are regarded by some as lymphangiomas,[54] but others think their spectrum of presentation is contiguous with that of purely venous abnormalities. They think that the term "orbital venous anomalies" should encompass both groups, particularly because the deep orbit does not contain lymphatics from which these lesions can arise.[52,55] Practically speaking, many of these lesions contain blood and phleboliths, both of which would suggest an incorporated venous component.[50,52]

Cause, Contributory Factors, Risk Factors

A 24-year review of 158 patients presenting with orbital venous anomalies found that 43% of patients presented before age 6, and 60% before age 16. About 43% of lesions involved the conjunctiva or sclera.[52] Other authors suggest that as many as 90% of lymphatic malformations are diagnosed by age 2.[56] Lesions are usually located in the head and neck region and can involve the orbit, eyelids, and conjunctiva. They comprise 0.3% to 1.5% of histopathologically diagnosed orbital tumors.[49] Some reports suggest a slight female predominance.[49,52]

Sequelae of the Problem

In general, ocular sequelae of lymphangiomas can be very similar to those of orbital hemangiomas. In children still at risk for amblyopia (younger than age 8), proptosis, motility restriction, and obstruction of the visual axis should trigger prompt referral to an ophthalmologist. It is important to remember that proptosis of the globe, when severe, can also cause injury to the optic nerve (and subsequent permanent vision loss) in a patient of any age. It has been noted that recurrent hemorrhages are common.[52]

Clinical Assessment

The most common presenting complaints in patients with orbital lymphangiomas are mass effect (42%), hemorrhage (37% at presentation and 55% in follow-up), ocular motility changes (28%), proptosis (15%), and decreased vision (8%).[52] Pain is often associated with hemorrhage. On examination, about 60% of patients had some degree of proptosis, whether they noticed it themselves or not.[52] The lesions do tend to enlarge slowly over time as the patient grows, but hemorrhage can precipitate sudden and dramatic enlargement.

Care must be taken to rule out more ominous entities in the differential diagnosis of lymphangiomas, including rhabdomyosarcomas and neuroblastomas. The imaging modality of choice for lymphangiomas is MRI. Lesions containing proteinaceous fluid will be best seen on T1-weighted images as well as T2-weighted images with fat saturation, whereas lesions containing blood are best seen on fat-saturated T1-weighted images. However, blood-containing structures may be confused with saturated fat on T2-weighted fat-saturated images. Contrast enhancement does not offer additional information in most cases, but can help to delineate venous components and solid vascular components.[10]

CT scanning provides less optimal soft tissue details and does involve radiation. However, when a scan is needed quickly, particularly in younger patients with contraindications to sedation, or in patients for whom imaging during Valsalva maneuver is desired, it can be a useful test.[10]

Management

Direct surgical excision of orbital lymphangiomas, although historically the standard treatment, can be problematic. Often, more than one procedure is needed.[57] The lesions tend to arborize with surrounding tissues, and surgical entry of the orbit itself is fraught with the potential to injure important structures such as the ophthalmic artery and its branches as well as several cranial nerves and their branches.[52] Extraconal (outside the muscle cone of the eye) and well-delineated lesions can be resected completely, but many lesions including intraconal and those with diffuse distributions must be resected in subtotal fashion. If complete resection is achieved, prognosis for short-term follow-up is excellent.[49] Nevertheless, several investigators recommend a conservative approach to treatment.[47,52,58]

In light of the difficulties with surgical resection, intralesional sclerosing therapy techniques for macrocystic lesions have also been described.[50,57,59,60] Most of these approaches are described on a small series of patients, and the protocols are variable.

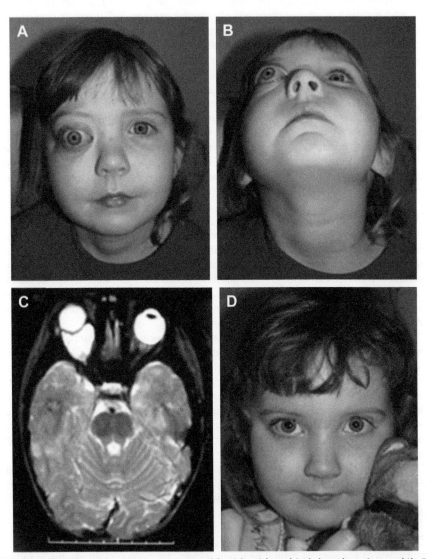

Fig. 4. Orbital lymphangioma. A 4-year-old girl with orbital lymphangioma. (*A*) Properrative presentation with proptosis and poor eyelid closure leading to ocular surface breakdown because of exposure. (*B*) Worm's eye view of the same patient, highlighting the proptosis. (*C*) T2-weighted MRI image demonstrating enhancing lesion occupying nearly the entire right orbit. (*D*) Same patient several months after 2 sessions of dual-drug percutaneous sclerotherapy.

Agents used have included tissue glue[59] and sodium morrhuate 5%[60] with some successful outcomes. Techniques include drainage of cysts followed by injection of sclerosing agent or tissue glue. A dual-drug technique has also been developed using sodium tetradecyl sulfate 3% and ethanol 98% for percutaneous sclerotherapy of lymphatic malformations in the orbit with good results (**Fig. 4**).[50,57] In addition, successful ablation of microcystic lesions using doxycycline foam has been reported.[50,57] Techniques such as these should be performed by, or in conjunction with, an interventional radiologist.

REFERENCES

1. Yap EY, Bartley GB, Hohberger GG. Periocular capillary hemangioma: a review for pediatricians and family physicians. Mayo Clin Proc 1998;73(8):753–9.
2. Kilcline C, Frieden IJ. Infantile hemangiomas: how common are they? A systematic review of the medical literature. Pediatr Dermatol 2008;25(2):168–73.
3. Günalp I, Gündüz K. Vascular tumors of the orbit. Doc Ophthalmol 1995;89(4): 337–45.
4. Drolet BA, Esterly NB, Frieden IJ. Hemangiomas in children. N Engl J Med 1999; 341(3):173–81.
5. Haggstrom AN, Drolet BA, Baselga E, et al. Prospective study of infantile hemangiomas: clinical characteristics predicting complications and treatment. Pediatrics 2006;118(3):882–7.
6. Jacobs AH, Walton RG. The incidence of birthmarks in the neonate. Pediatrics 1976;58(2):218–22.
7. Haik BG, Karcioglu ZA, Gordon RA, et al. Capillary hemangioma (infantile periocular hemangioma). Surv Ophthalmol 1994;38(5):399–426.
8. Hartzell LD, Buckmiller LM. Current management of infantile hemangiomas and their common associated conditions. Otolaryngol Clin North Am 2012;45(3): 545–56.
9. Chang LC, Haggstrom AN, Drolet BA, et al. Growth characteristics of infantile hemangiomas: implications for management. Pediatrics 2008;122(2):360–7.
10. Bilaniuk LT. Vascular lesions of the orbit in children. Neuroimaging Clin N Am 2012;15(1):107–20.
11. Hernandez JA, Chia A, Quah BL, et al. Periocular capillary hemangioma: management practices in recent years. Clin Ophthalmol 2013;7:1227–32.
12. Huoh KC, Rosbe KW. Infantile hemangiomas of the head and neck. Pediatr Clin North Am 2013;60(4):937–49.
13. Nasseri E, Piram M, McCuaig CC, et al. Partially involuting congenital hemangiomas: a report of 8 cases and review of the literature. J Am Acad Dermatol 2014;70(1):75–9.
14. Mulliken JB, Glowacki J. Hemangiomas and vascular malformations in infants and children: a classification based on endothelial characteristics. Plast Reconstr Surg 1982;69(3):412–22.
15. Takahashi K, Mulliken JB, Kozakewich HP, et al. Cellular markers that distinguish the phases of hemangioma during infancy and childhood. J Clin Invest 1994; 93(6):2357–64.
16. Haggstrom AN, Drolet BA, Baselga E, et al. Prospective study of infantile hemangiomas: demographic, prenatal, and perinatal characteristics. J Pediatr 2007; 150:291–4.
17. Glowacki J, Mulliken JB. Mast cells in hemangiomas and vascular malformations. Pediatrics 1982;70(1):48–51.

18. Kleinman ME, Greives MR, Churgin SS, et al. Hypoxia-induced mediators of stem/progenitor cell trafficking are increased in children with hemangioma. Arterioscler Thromb Vasc Biol 2007;27(12):2664–70.
19. Stigmar G, Crawford JS, Ward CM, et al. Ophthalmic sequelae of infantile hemangiomas of the eyelids and orbit. Am J Ophthalmol 1978;85(6):806–13.
20. Haik BG, Jakobiec FA, Ellsworth RM, et al. Capillary hemangioma of the lids and orbit: an analysis of the clinical features and therapeutic results in 101 cases. Ophthalmology 1979;86(5):760–92.
21. Frieden IJ, Haggstrom AN, Drolet BA, et al. Infantile hemangiomas: current knowledge, future directions. Proceedings of a research workshop on infantile hemangiomas, April 7-9, 2005, Bethesda, Maryland, USA. Pediatr Dermatol 2005;22(5):383–406.
22. Horii KA, Drolet BA, Frieden IJ. Prospective study of the frequency of hepatic hemangiomas in infants with multiple cutaneous infantile hemangiomas. Pediatr Dermatol 2011;28(3):245–53.
23. Kasabach HH, Merritt KK. Capillary hemangioma with extensive purpura: report of a case. Am J Dis Child 1940;59:1063–70.
24. Hall GW. Kasabach-Merritt syndrome: pathogenesis and management. Br J Haematol 2001;112(4):851–62.
25. Metry D, Heyer G, Hess C, et al. Consensus statement on diagnostic criteria for PHACE syndrome. Pediatrics 2009;124(5):1447–56.
26. Metry D, Frieden IJ, Hess C, et al. Propranolol use in PHACE syndrome with cervical and intracranial arterial anomalies: collective experience in 32 infants. Pediatr Dermatol 2013;30(1):71–89.
27. Zarem HA, Edgerton MT. Induced resolution of cavernous hemangiomas following prednisolone therapy. Plast Reconstr Surg 1967;39(1):76–83.
28. De Venecia G, Lobeck CC. Successful treatment of eyelid hemangioma with prednisone. Arch Ophthalmol 1970;84(1):98–102.
29. Fost NC, Esterly NB. Successful treatment of juvenile hemangiomas with prednisone. J Pediatr 1968;72(3):351–7.
30. Hiles DA, Pilchard WA. Corticosteroid control of neonatal hemangiomas of the orbit and ocular adnexa. Am J Ophthalmol 1971;71(5):1003–8.
31. Ruttum MS, Abrams GW, Harris GJ, et al. Bilateral retinal embolization associated with intralesional corticosteroid injection for capillary hemangioma of infancy. J Pediatr Ophthalmol Strabismus 1993;30(1):4–7.
32. Shorr N, Seiff SR. Central retinal artery occlusion associated with periocular corticosteroid injection for juvenile hemangioma. Ophthalmic Surg 1986;17(4):229–31.
33. Plager DA, Snyder SK. Resolution of astigmatism after surgical resection of capillary hemangiomas in infants. Ophthalmology 1997;104(7):1102–6.
34. Deans RM, Harris GJ, Kivlin JD. Surgical dissection of capillary hemangiomas. An alternative to intralesional corticosteroids. Arch Ophthalmol 1992;110(12):1743–7.
35. Walker RS, Custer PL, Nerad JA. Surgical excision of periorbital capillary hemangiomas. Ophthalmology 1994;101(8):1333–40.
36. Léauté-Labrèze C, Dumas de la Roque E, Hubiche T, et al. Propranolol for severe hemangiomas of infancy. N Engl J Med 2008;358(24):2649–51.
37. Drolet BA, Frommelt PC, Chamlin SL, et al. Initiation and use of propranolol for infantile hemangioma: report of a consensus conference. Pediatrics 2013;131(1):128–40.
38. Gomulka J, Siegel DH, Drolet BA. Dramatic shift in the infantile hemangioma treatment paradigm at a single institution. Pediatr Dermatol 2013;30(6):751–2.

39. Guo S, Ni N. Topical treatment for capillary hemangioma of the eyelid using beta-blocker solution. Arch Ophthalmol 2010;128(2):255-6.
40. Yu L, Li S, Su B, et al. Treatment of superficial infantile hemangiomas with timolol: evaluation of short-term efficacy and safety in infants. Exp Ther Med 2013;6(2): 388-90.
41. Chambers CB, Katowitz WR, Katowitz JA, et al. A controlled study of topical 0.25% timolol maleate gel for the treatment of cutaneous infantile capillary hemangiomas. Ophthal Plast Reconstr Surg 2012;28(2):103-6.
42. Ni N, Langer P, Wagner R, et al. Topical timolol for periocularhemangioma: report of further study. Arch Ophthalmol 2011;129(3):377-9.
43. Khunger N, Pahwa M. Dramatic response to topical timolol lotion of a large hemifacial infantile haemangioma associated with PHACE syndrome. Br J Dermatol 2011;164(4):886-8.
44. Pope E, Chakkittakandiyil A. Topical timolol gel for infantile hemangiomas: a pilot study. Arch Dermatol 2010;146(5):564-5.
45. Tanner JL, Dechert MP, Frieden IJ. Growing up with a facial hemangioma: parent and child coping and adaptation. Pediatrics 1998;101(3 Pt 1):446-52.
46. Frieden IJ, Eichenfield LF, Esterly NB, et al. Guidelines of care for hemangiomas of infancy. American Academy of Dermatology Guidelines/Outcomes Committee. J Am Acad Dermatol 1997;37(4):631-7.
47. Chung EM, Smirniotopoulos JG, Specht CS, et al. From the archives of the AFIP: pediatric orbit tumors and tumorlike lesions: nonosseous lesions of the extraocular orbit. Radiographics 2007;27(6):1777-99.
48. Iliff WJ, Green WR. Orbital lymphangiomas. Ophthalmology 1979;86(5):914-29.
49. Gündüz K, Demirel S, Yagmurlu B, et al. Correlation of surgical outcome with neuroimaging findings in periocular lymphangiomas. Ophthalmology 2006; 113(7):1231.e1-8.
50. Hill RH 3rd, Shiels WE 2nd, Foster JA, et al. Percutaneous drainage and ablation as first line therapy for macrocystic and microcystic orbital lymphatic malformations. Ophthal Plast Reconstr Surg 2012;28(2):119-25.
51. Rootman J, Hay E, Graeb D, et al. Orbital-adnexal lymphangiomas. A spectrum of hemodynamically isolated vascular hamartomas. Ophthalmology 1986; 93(12):1558-70.
52. Wright JE, Sullivan TJ, Garner A, et al. Orbital venous anomalies. Ophthalmology 1997;104(6):905-13.
53. Harris GJ. Orbital vascular malformations: a consensus statement on terminology and its clinical implications. Orbital Society. Am J Ophthalmol 1999;127(4):453-5.
54. Jones IS. Lymphangiomas of the ocular adnexa: an analysis of 62 cases. Trans Am Ophthalmol Soc 1959;57:602-65.
55. Wright JE. Orbital vascular anomalies. Trans Am Acad Ophthalmol Otolaryngol 1974;78(4):606-16.
56. Giguère CM, Bauman NM, Smith RJ. New treatment options for lymphangioma in infants and children. Ann Otol Rhinol Laryngol 2002;111(12 Pt 1):1066-75.
57. Shiels WE 2nd, Kang DR, Murakami JW, et al. Percutaneous treatment of lymphatic malformations. Otolaryngol Head Neck Surg 2009;141(2):219-24.
58. Schick U, Hassler W. Treatment of deep vascular orbital malformations. Clin Neurol Neurosurg 2009;111(10):801-7.
59. Hayasaki A, Nakamura H, Hamasaki T, et al. Successful treatment of intraorbital lymphangioma with tissue fibrin glue. Surg Neurol 2009;72(6):722-4.
60. Schwarcz RM, Ben Simon GJ, Cook T, et al. Sclerosing therapy as first line treatment for low flow vascular lesions of the orbit. Am J Ophthalmol 2006;141(2):333-9.

Genetics and Ocular Disorders: A Focused Review

Hannah L. Scanga, MS, CGC[a,b], Ken K. Nischal, MD, FRCOphth[a,b],*

KEYWORDS

- Eye disease • Genetics • Genetic testing • Pediatrics

KEY POINTS

- Increasingly accurate phenotyping leads to better genetic evaluation.
- Genetic eye conditions may be due to a common cellar defect (eg, ciliopathies or RASopathies).
- Early-onset retinal dystrophies may be associated with renal disease.
- An understanding of genetic testing helps clinicians identify shortcomings in testing which may lead to a better understanding of the most appropriate test for a given ocular condition.
- Dedicated genetic counselors within ophthalmic and pediatric clinics are likely to improve the delivery of clinical care in these settings.

INTRODUCTION

Genetic eye disease is a vast topic. So many areas of interest exist and so many enormous developments have occurred that providing a comprehensive discussion in a short review such as this is impossible. Therefore, this article concentrates on some new concepts in ophthalmic genetics, and also provides some strategies that may help pediatricians cope with all of the new information in the world of genomics. This article also helps identify patients who might benefit from genetic evaluation and provides some idea of how to interpret those genetic results.

The pediatrician and ophthalmologist often work as a team to determine a diagnosis to account for all physical and developmental anomalies that might present in a child. Whenever concern exists about a child's development, it is important for an ophthalmologist to conduct an evaluation to assess vision and possible related eye anomalies.

The newborn screening examination and the family ocular history provide critical information to pediatricians. Any anatomic anomaly seen by the pediatrician might indicate a genetic disease, which might impact not only the child's vision but also the

[a] UPMC Eye Center, University of Pittsburgh, 200 Lothrop Street, Pittsburgh, PA 15213, USA;
[b] Children's Eye Center, Children's Hospital of Pittsburgh of UPMC, 4401 Penn Avenue, Pittsburgh, PA 15224-1334, USA
* Corresponding author. Children's Hospital of Pittsburgh, CHL 03-05-01, 4401 Penn Avenue, Pittsburgh, PA 15224-1334.
E-mail address: nischalkk@upmc.edu

Pediatr Clin N Am 61 (2014) 555–565
http://dx.doi.org/10.1016/j.pcl.2014.03.005
0031-3955/14/$ – see front matter © 2014 Elsevier Inc. All rights reserved.
pediatric.theclinics.com

overall health of the child. For example, a lens opacity could represent galactosemia. Conversely, if a history exists of a genetic eye defect, the baby should have an immediate thorough evaluation. For example, a family might have a history of incontinentia pigmenti. This disease can variably affect the retinas of different people. A mother might have normal vision, but her child could inherit a form of the disease that will cause blindness if treatment is not obtained before the retinas detach. Therefore, the pediatrician can help prevent total loss of vision if a child with incontinentia pigmenti is referred immediately for retinal examination regardless of the parent's vision.

SELECTED CLINICALLY IMPORTANT OCULAR PHENOTYPE/GENOTYPE CORRELATIONS

This section presents either recent information that is important to know or older information that is still so important that it needs to be revisited.

Lids

Lymphedema-distichiasis syndrome
This syndrome is caused by mutations in FOXC2 and has significant variability of expression.[1] Distichiasis (the growth of extra eyelashes, ranging from a few extra eyelashes to a full extra set on both the upper and lower lids) is the most common clinical feature, followed by lymphedema, which typically has its onset at puberty and not at birth (Milroy disease). Therefore, any child with distichiasis should be genetically tested for this condition.

Cornea

Corneal lesion and trisomy 8 mosaicism
Corneal lesions present as a flat reticular-appearing white lesion usually extending from the limbus into the cornea; fine blood vessels are usually present and the lesion is not elevated (**Fig. 1**).[2] This lesion is most commonly seen in trisomy 8 mosaicism, and the affected child may seem normal, and therefore testing (see later discussion) should be considered.

Iris

Iris anomalies and ACTA2
Cysts from the iris pigment epithelium at the pupillary margin are also called *iris flocculi* (**Fig. 2**). If a patient has parents or siblings with the same condition or has a family history of cardiac problems or vascular dissection, then ACTA2 analysis should be considered.[3] Congenital mydriasis with persistent pupillary membranes has also been found to be associated with ACTA2 mutations.[4]

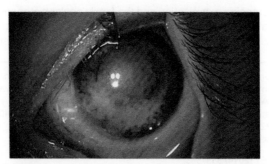

Fig. 1. This corneal lesion is unilateral; there is a flat reticular pattern with fine vessels. If seen, trisomy 8 mosaicism should be excluded.

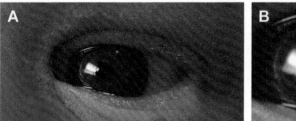
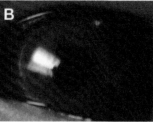

Fig. 2. This child has iris flocculi, which from a distance may appear like an irregular pupil (*A*), but close up the cysts of the iris pigment epithelium coming through the pupil are seen (*B*). A family history of these or of cardiovascular anomalies should prompt testing for ACTA2 mutations.

Lens

The relationship between intracerebral hemorrhages, in utero or perinatally, with congenital cataracts or lens anomalies has been found to be associated with mutations in the COL4A1 gene. This gene encodes the α1 chain of type IV collagen, which is a critical component of almost all basement membranes, including those of the vasculature, renal glomeruli, and ocular structures.[5]

Vitreous

Vitreous anomaly and stickler syndrome

Stickler syndrome is a collagenopathy caused by mutations in COL2A1 and COL11A1. Stickler syndrome consists of cleft palate, arthropathy, myopia, and retinal detachment. Ocular-only phenotype is seen in mutations in COL2A1. Some people argue that all patients with cleft palate should be screened for vitreous anomaly (**Fig. 3**).[6]

Retina

Leber congenital amaurosis

The number of gene mutations that are known to cause Leber congenital amaurosis (LCA) increases as the knowledge base increases, but the LCA genes encode proteins with a wide variety of retinal functions, such as phototransduction (AIPL1, GUCY2D), rod/cone morphogenesis (CRB1, CRX), vitamin A cycle regulation (LRAT, RDH12, RPE65), guanine synthesis (IMPDH1), outer segment phagocytosis (MERTK), and

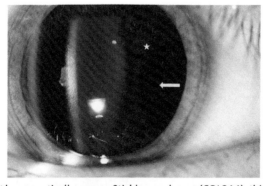

Fig. 3. This patient has genetically proven Stickler syndrome (COL2A1); this is a type 1 vitreous anomaly. Normally the area behind the membranous vitreous structure (*white star*) would reflect some light, but here it is optically empty (*white arrow*). (*Courtesy of* M. Snead, MD.)

intraphotoreceptor ciliary transport processes (ciliary genes: CEP290, LCA5, RPGRIP1, TULP1, discussed later).[7]

Phenotype-genotype correlation by one Hanein and colleagues[8] suggested that patients could be divided into 2 main groups, one with photophobia and the other with nyctalopia.

Photophobia

In the group complaining of photophobia, hypermetropia was always noted and involvement was seen of both rods and cones, resulting in early peripheral and macular degeneration of the retina with bone spicule pigments in the periphery; retinal atrophy including the macular region; thin attenuated vessels; and optic disc pallor. When the hypermetropia was higher than +7 diopters, the visual acuity was reduced to counting fingers (CF) or light perception (LP). In these cases, the disease was not progressive and pathognomonic of GUCY2D mutations when the hypermetropia was lower than +7; the visual acuity was frequently recordable and ranged from CF to 20/400. This findings, together with the presence of a keratoconus, suggested mutations in the AIPL1 or RPGRIP1 genes.

Nyctalopia

In the group with night blindness (nyctalopia), 2 clinical subtypes exist, one with hypermetropia and the second without hypermetropia. In the former, an early macular disruption is almost always visible on fundoscopy. Consequently, a central scotoma is noted at the visual field and the visual acuity ranges from 20/200 to 20/100 in the first decade of life. These clinical findings suggest mutations in either CRB1 or CRX. In the second subtype, an early peripheral pigmentary retinopathy is visible on fundoscopy. The visual field shows a progressive concentric reduction. The visual acuity is much better than in other groups of patients, especially during daytime, reaching values ranging from 20/200 to 20/100 or better during the first decade. This milder form of LCA strongly suggests mutations in the RPE65 or TULP1 genes.

Optic Nerve

Most inherited optic neuropathies are caused by mutations in mitochondrial DNA (Leber hereditary optic neuropathy LHON) or mutations in the nuclear gene OPA1 causing autosomal dominant optic (ADOA) neuropathy (Kjer's type) see **Fig. 4**. OPA1 encodes mitochondrial proteins but is in nuclear DNA. Mutations in mitochondrial

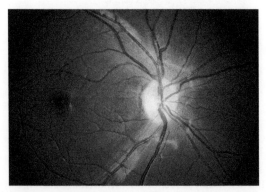

Fig. 4. This child has OPA1 positive mutation; this is autosomal dominant optic atrophy. Note the wedge shaped atrophy temporally.

DNA causing LHON are maternally inherited, whereas mutations in OPA1 are autosomal dominantly inherited from the mother or father. Clinical expressivity is so variable in both conditions that they can be difficult to differentiate unless the inheritance pattern is elucidated with an accurate pedigree. Patients with LHON may benefit from avoidance of certain environmental exposures (smoking, alcohol consumption) that may cause deterioration of the disease. Furthermore, because both diseases (LHON and ADOA) are mitochondrial dysfunctions, an over-the-counter supplement, idebenone, which reduces "stress" on mitochondria, has been shown to have a protective effect in both diseases.[9-11]

Glaucoma

Mutations in 6 genes (MYOC, PITX2, FOXC1, PAX6, CYP1B1, and LTBP2) are known to cause early-onset glaucoma.[12] Mutations in CYP1B1 and LTBP2 are the only ones that cause recessive disease, whereas the remainder cause glaucoma in a dominant manner. Furthermore, individuals with early-onset glaucoma caused by mutations in MYOC coding for myocilin may be treated in the future with agents that minimize the effects of endoplasmic reticulum stress or may be eligible for clinical trials to test new topical drugs.[13]

DEVELOPMENT OF GROUPINGS OF DISEASES AND SYNDROMES BASED ON CELLULAR EVENTS OR PATHWAYS
Ciliopathies

Two types of cilia exist: intracellular cilia and motile cilia. Intracellular cilia are complex sensory organelles involved in the control of a variety of cellular signaling pathways. These cilia are highly conserved throughout evolution. Cilia receive a variety of extracellular signals, which they transduce and thereby affect proliferation, nerve growth, polarity, differentiation, or tissue maintenance. Since cilia are in all cells, mutations in genes coding for components of cilia affect a multitude of tissues and organ systems in which the cilium-centromere complex functions are important. Ciliopathies are a genetically heterogeneous group of disorders caused by mutations in genes whose products localize to the cilium–centrosome complex.[14,15]

Important examples of ciliopathies are as follows:

- Retinal-renal syndrome (eg, Senior-Loken syndrome): nephronophthisis in association with retinal dystrophy. Retinal dystrophies are not present in every form of nephronophthisis, but the chance increases if mutations in nephrocystin-5 (NPHP5) are present. NPHP5 interacts with RPGR (mutations in this can cause isolated X-linked retinitis pigmentosa), and both genes are localized in the cilia of renal epithelial cells and retinal photoreceptors, respectively (**Fig. 5**).
- Joubert syndrome: consists of developmental delay and ataxia caused by hypoplasia of the cerebellar vermis in association with retinal coloboma, and is characterized by an irregular breathing pattern during the neonatal period. Recessive mutations in NPHP3, NPHP6/CEP290, NPHP8/RPGRIP1L, AHI1, MKS3, ARL13B, INPP5E, and TMEM216, and NPHP1 deletions cause Joubert syndrome.[15]
- Meckel syndrome: an autosomal recessive disease that results in perinatal death from dysplasia and malformation of multiple organs. It is characterized by occipital meningoencephalocele, microphthalmia, lung hypoplasia, polycystic kidneys, or renal dysplasia, biliary ectasia, postaxial polydactyly, and situs inversus. Mutations have been described in MKS1, MKS3, NPHP3, NPHP6/CEP290, NPHP8/RPGRIP1L, TMEM216, and CC2D2A.

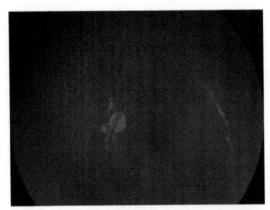

Fig. 5. This child with early-onset retinal dystrophy (age <1 year) was found to have polydipsia and polyuria associated with renal tubular injury/nephronophthisis on evaluation by the renal team.

- Bardet-Biedl syndrome: the Bardet-Biedl syndrome is a multisystem disorder characterized by retinal degeneration, cystic kidney disease, developmental delay, diabetes mellitus, obesity, infertility, and postaxial polydactyly. Mutations in 16 genes (BBS1 to BBS12, MKS1, NPHP6/CEP290, SDCCAG8, and SEPT7 [septin 7]) can cause the Bardet-Biedl syndrome phenotype.
- Usher syndrome: ten different genes are associated with this deaf/blind condition. These genes encode several structurally and functionally distinct proteins, which play a role in stereocilia development in cochlear hair cells, explaining the deafness phenotype when these molecular interactions are perturbed. The mystery is that photoreceptors lack a similar apparatus, and therefore a common theory has been missing for Usher protein function in the 2 neurosensory cell types affected in this syndrome. However, recent animal model work suggests that Usher proteins might regulate protein trafficking between the inner and outer segments of photoreceptors.[16]
- Some retinal dystrophy genes are also known to be ciliary genes, such as RP1, RPGR, and RPGRIP1. At present, they do not appear to affect other organ systems.

The severity and extent of organ involvement in ciliopathies depend on the following mechanisms:

- Specific gene mutations cause specific phenotypes. For example, homozygous deletions of NPHP1 usually cause nephronophthisis, whereas 2 truncating mutations of NPHP6/CEP290 cause a Meckel-type phenotype, which is more severe.
- The type of mutation affects phenotype. For example, 2 truncating mutations of NPHP3, NPHP6, NPHP8, or NPHP11/MKS380 cause Meckel syndrome, but the presence of even one missense mutation may result in a milder form of Joubert syndrome.
- Modifier genes affect phenotype. For example, in patients with homozygous NPHP1 deletions (renal only), the presence of an additional heterozygous mutation in NPHP6 or NPHP8 causes additional eye or cerebellar involvement (retinal dystrophy or Joubert syndrome).
- Oligogenicity affects phenotype. For example, Bardet-Biedl syndrome may be caused by the interaction of 2 or more recessive genes with heterozygous

mutations (which would not result in disease themselves because the mutations are not homozygous).

Motile cilia are structurally similar to primary cilia. Genetic defects of these cause primary ciliary dyskinesia, such as Kartagener disease.

RASopathies

The term *RASopathies* refers to a group of 5 neurodevelopmental syndromes (Noonan, LEOPARD, Costello, Cardiofaciocutaneous, and neurofibromatosis-Noonan syndrome) caused by mutations in genes encoding proteins involved in the RAS/MAPK (rat sarcoma/mitogen-activated protein kinase) signaling pathway. This pathway plays a role in regulation of cell determination, proliferation, differentiation, migration, and senescence, and disruption of this pathway can lead to the risk of tumorigenesis and, some evidence suggests, abnormal healing. The study of RASopathies is in its infancy.[17]

OVERVIEW OF GENETIC TESTING AND PRINCIPLES

This section reviews the capabilities, benefits, and limitations of common genetic testing that may be used in the diagnosis of various ophthalmic conditions. A summary was recently published of the methods used in the select tests discussed herein, with special focus on inherited eye diseases.[18,19]

Karyotype

Karyotyping is the traditional cytogenetic method used for the assessment of chromosome number and structure. The chromosomal complement is assessed through microscopy. Anomalies are described following the International System for Human Cytogenetic Nomenclature (ISCN), last updated in 2013.[1] Specifically, the resolution of a karyotype is limited to visible alterations, wherein the smallest detectable abnormality is approximately 5 megabases (Mb). Any abnormality below this level will not be observed, resulting in a normal karyotype.

Furthermore, a karyotype may not demonstrate mosaicism, a state in which an individual carries 2 or more genetically distinct cell lines. Because the proportion of mosaic cells may differ among tissues, the likelihood of detecting mosaicism increases with the number of cells counted and, potentially, the sampled tissue. In cases of suspected mosaicism, the number of cells assessed should be increased, from a minimum of 5 in a traditional karyotype to at least 25 or 50 cells.[20]

For the ophthalmologist, karyotype is most likely to be encountered in the setting of a family history of a chromosome abnormality, individuals in whom a particular chromosome abnormality is suspected based on phenotype, or cases of multiple congenital anomalies for which a specific syndrome is not yet obvious. In summary, the diagnostic utility of chromosome analysis is limited to monosomies, trisomies, balanced and unbalanced translocations, and microdeletion and microduplication syndromes.

Microarray-Based Technologies

Microarrays are cytogenetically based tests focusing on detecting copy number variations in specific alleles across the genome. A *copy number variant* is defined as a genomic segment of at least 1000 nucleotide bases that differ in number when compared with reference genomes.[21]

The 2 major types of microarrays, comparative genomic hybridization (CGH) and single nucleotide polymorphism (SNP) arrays, are discussed later. Comparative genomic hybridization arrays detect copy number variations by using oligonucleotides (small, synthetic DNA fragments) that correspond to specific chromosomal loci. Targeted CGH arrays may limit the loci to only those associated with genetic disorders, whereas other CGH arrays are more comprehensive. Differences in hybridization intensity between the patient's DNA sample and a reference DNA sample indicate the presence of a copy number variant.[22] Comparative genomic hybridization arrays are only capable of detecting changes in copy number, specifically, monosomies, trisomies, unbalanced chromosome translocations, microdeletions, and microduplications at chromosomal loci covered by the oligonucleotide probes. Most notably, CGH arrays are unable to detect balanced chromosome translocations, which would be apparent on a karyotype.

Single nucleotide polymorphism arrays use known polymorphic markers in the human genome to detect copy-number and copy number–neutral variations in the genome. Similar to CGH arrays, the hybridization intensity of the patient's sample to the test probes can quantify the relative amount of DNA present for individual SNPs. Single nucleotide polymorphism arrays are often combined with CGH array technologies, enhancing the diagnostic yield. Compared with karyotyping, the resolutions of microarrays can be less than 100 kilobases.

Comparative genomic hybridization and SNP arrays are used in a pediatric setting for cases involving developmental delay, intellectual disability, or multiple congenital anomalies. A microarray is often a first-line genetic test when a patient's phenotype does not yet suggest a specific genetic syndrome and a detection level greater than karyotyping is desired. Not all copy number variants are pathogenic, and variants of uncertain significance are frequently encountered.[23]

Sequencing

DNA sequencing is a primer-initiated technology that allows the sequence of specific genes to be assessed and compared with a reference sequence. Sequencing detects mutations affecting a single nucleotide or a short run of consecutive nucleotides. More specifically, missense, nonsense, frameshift, and splice site mutations are detected by sequencing, as are small insertions and deletions.

The yield of DNA sequencing depends on multiple factors. First, the sensitivity of DNA sequencing is high, but is ultimately depends on the appropriateness of the test given the clinical presentation. Second, a particular condition may be the result of one of several genes, some of which have yet to be recognized as having a role in the pathogenesis of certain diseases. Only the genes known to have this role can be tested, leaving a proportion of cases without a known molecular cause. Third, repetitive sequences within tested genes may limit the areas assessed or the interpretation. This is caused by "slippage" during sequencing, wherein the polymerase cannot accurately bind to the template sequence because of the repetitiveness of the region. Finally, methodologies vary among laboratories with regard to whether all coding exons are sequenced and whether the intronic sequences are included. Furthermore, mutations upstream or downstream from the targeted gene may affect gene expression and are not routinely assessed by commercial laboratories.

In ophthalmologic diseases, sequencing is most useful when a clinical diagnosis is associated with mutations in one or a few genes. As genetic research and technologies expand, knowledge about the relationships between genes and phenotypes increases and the cost of sequencing is decreases, making single-gene studies less relevant for certain diagnoses. To counteract this, DNA sequencing can be performed for numerous genes at one time, such as in a condition-specific panel or in exome sequencing.

Condition-specific panels target the known genes associated with a particular ophthalmic condition, whereas exome sequencing covers approximately 95% of the coding regions of genome. Given the complexities of exome sequencing and the vast amount of information it can provide, both related and unrelated to an individual's symptoms, it is prudent to involve a genetics professional for this testing.

Deletion/Duplication Studies

Deletion/duplication studies use a variety of methods to detect imbalances within a specific gene. In general, these studies complement DNA sequencing in that they are capable of detecting deletions or duplications that may be missed by direct sequencing. These may be missed because DNA sequencing is only able to detect variations compared with a known sequence and has no mechanism for detecting copy number.

DNA sequencing is initiated by primers, which hybridize to the DNA and allow the reaction to proceed. In the presence of a deletion of one of the 2 alleles, the primer is able to hybridize to the intact copy and generate the sequence. Therefore, the test still has an output, and the absence of 1 allele goes undetected. In the presence of a duplication, the primer is able to hybridize to all copies of the allele, allowing the reaction to proceed normally. Because both deletions and duplications of partial or entire genes may account for the pathogenesis of a condition, these variations may be undetected by DNA sequencing, and an individual's molecular diagnosis may not be fully achieved.

The utility of deletion/duplication studies varies, depending on the proportion of cases of a particular disease attributed to copy number variations at the gene level, and the laboratory methods used. Today, one of the most widely used methods is multiplex ligation-dependent probe amplification (MLPA). Multiplex ligation-dependent probe amplification uses probes throughout a targeted DNA sequence. When the probe's sequence is present in the test sample, hybridization and amplification of the probe itself occurs. The amount of the probe is then quantified and the relative amount of the targeted sequences can be determined. In the case of deletions and duplications, fewer and more probes will be detected, respectively. Depending on the size of a gene, MLPA can assess changes to copy number at an exon level.

For clinicians, deletion/duplication studies should be considered when a high clinical suspicion exists for a genetic disease and DNA sequencing was normal. Modern sequencing methods "read" the sequence like a book and see if "it makes sense"; if a whole sentence was missing as the book is "read," one may not realize that anything was wrong as long as the preceding sentence and the following sentence still "flow". This fact is particularly relevant for conditions in which changes to copy number are recognized causes of the disorder. Deletion/duplication studies are irrelevant for men with X-linked conditions, because primers used in DNA sequencing would fail to hybridize to a deleted sequence and no second X chromosome is present to mask the aberration.

NEW THERAPIES FOR GENETIC EYE DISEASE

Much work is in progress at ex vivo and animal model levels for gene therapies for various parts of the eye, including the cornea, trabecular meshwork, and optic nerve, but the area of most advancement in human clinical trials is the treatment of some retinal dystrophies. Specifically, patients with LCA are being treated with gene therapy, but only patients with LCA and mutations in RPE65 can potentially benefit from current RPE65 gene-based clinical trials. Before considering this therapy, a molecular diagnosis must be established using a genetic test. Recently, 3 clinical trials of gene therapy using recombinant adeno-associated virus vectors have been reported for the treatment of RPE65-related LCA. Substantial gains in visual function of clinical trial participants provide evidence for relevant biologic activity resulting from a newly introduced gene. Reviews of these groundbreaking findings have been published elsewhere.[24,25]

Recently a group[26] reported preliminary results of gene therapy in 6 men with choroideremia; the 6-month results show promising signs of visual improvement.

SUMMARY

To ensure that patients have the best access to the latest therapies, pediatric ophthalmologists and pediatricians must be receptive to the signs and symptoms of genetic eye disease. Molecular testing should be undertaken with the help of a genetic counselor and/or geneticist. Some academic centers have access to genetic counselors with expertise in ophthalmic genetic disorders, and these experts are invaluable in helping to direct testing and counseling.

REFERENCES

1. Allen RC. Genetic diseases affecting the eyelids: what should a clinician know? Curr Opin Ophthalmol 2013;24(5):463–77.
2. Mataftsi A, Islam L, Kelberman D, et al. Chromosome abnormalities and the genetics of congenital corneal opacification. Mol Vis 2011;17:1624–40.
3. Chamney S, McGimpsey S, McConnell V, et al. Iris flocculi as an ocular marker of ACTA2 mutation in familial thoracic aortic aneurysms and dissections. Ophthalmic Genet 2013. [Epub ahead of print].
4. Moller HU, Fledelius HC, Milewicz DM, et al. Eye features in three Danish patients with multisystemic smooth muscle dysfunction syndrome. Br J Ophthalmol 2012; 96(9):1227–31.
5. Colin E, Sentilhes L, Sarfati A, et al. Fetal intracerebral hemorrhage and cataract: think COL4A1. J Perinatol 2014;34(1):75–7.
6. Snead MP, McNinch AM, Poulson AV, et al. Richards Stickler syndrome, ocular-only variants and a key diagnostic role for the ophthalmologist. Eye (Lond) 2011;25:1389–400.
7. den Hollander AI, Roepman R, Koenekoop RK, et al. Leber congenital amaurosis: genes, proteins and disease mechanisms. Prog Retin Eye Res 2008;27(4): 391–419.
8. Hanein S, Perrault I, Gerber S, et al. Leber congenital amaurosis: comprehensive survey of the genetic heterogeneity, refinement of the clinical definition, and genotype-phenotype correlations as a strategy for molecular diagnosis. Hum Mutat 2004;23(4):306–17.
9. Barboni P, Valentino ML, La Morgia C, et al. Idebenone treatment in patients with OPA1-mutant dominant optic atrophy. Brain 2013;136(Pt 2):e231.
10. Rudolph G, Dimitriadis K, Büchner B, et al. Effects of idebenone on color vision in patients with leber hereditary optic neuropathy. J Neuroophthalmol 2013;33(1): 30–6.
11. Yu-Wai-Man P, Griffiths PG, Chinnery PF. Mitochondrial optic neuropathies: disease mechanisms and therapeutic strategies. Prog Retin Eye Res 2011;30(2): 81–114.
12. Fan BJ, Wiggs JL. Glaucoma: genes, phenotypes, and new directions for therapy. J Clin Invest 2010;120(9):3064–72.

13. Zode GS, Bugge KE, Mohan K, et al. Topical ocular sodium 4-phenylbutyrate rescues glaucoma in a myocilin mouse model of primary open-angle glaucoma. Invest Ophthalmol Vis Sci 2012;53(3):1557–65.
14. Adams NA, Awadein A, Toma HS. The retinal ciliopathies. Ophthalmic Genet 2007;28:113–25.
15. Hildebrandt F, Benzing T, Katsanis N. Ciliopathies. N Engl J Med 2011;364: 1533–43.
16. Cosgrove D, Zallocchi M. Usher protein functions in hair cells and photoreceptors. Int J Biochem Cell Biol 2014;46:80–9.
17. Cizmarova M, Kostalova L, Pribilincova Z, et al. Rasopathies—dysmorphic syndromes with short stature and risk of malignancy. Endocr Regul 2013;47:217–22.
18. Gabriel LA, Traboulsi EI. Genetic diagnostic methods for inherited eye disease. Middle East Afr J Ophthalmol 2011;18(1):24–9.
19. Shaffer LG, McGowan-Jordan J, Schmid M, editors. An international system for human cytogenetic nomenclature. Unionville (CT): S. Karger Publishers, Inc; 2013.
20. Scott SA, Cohen N, Brandt T, et al. Detection of low-level mosaicism and placental mosaicism by oligonucelotide array comparative genomic hybridization. Genet Med 2010;12:85–92.
21. Feuk L, Carson AR, Scherer SW. Structural variation in the human genome. Nat Rev Genet 2006;7(2):85–97.
22. Oostlander AE, Meijer GA, Ylstra B. Microarray-based comparative genomic hybridization and its application in human genetics. Clin Genet 2004;66:488–95.
23. Manning M, Louanne H. Array-based technology and recommendations for utilization in medical genetics practice for detection of chromosomal abnormalities. Genet Med 2010;12(11):742–5.
24. Cideciyan AV. Leber congenital amaurosis due to *RPE65* mutations and its treatment with gene therapy. Prog Retin Eye Res 2010;29(5):398–427.
25. Jacobson SG, Cideciyan AV, Ratnakaram R, et al. Gene therapy for Leber congenital amaurosis caused by RPE65 mutations: safety and efficacy in 15 children and adults followed up to 3 years. Arch Ophthalmol 2012;130(1):9–24.
26. MacLaren RE, Groppe M, Barnard AR, et al. Retinal gene therapy in patients with choroideremia: initial findings from a phase 1/2 clinical trial. Lancet 2014. http://dx.doi.org/10.1016/S0140-6736(13)62117-0.

Retinopathy of Prematurity

Catherine O. Jordan, MD

KEYWORDS

- Retinopathy of prematurity (ROP) • Retrolental fibroplasia
- Vascular endothelial growth factor inhibitors • Prematurity • Low birth weight

KEY POINTS

- Supplemental oxygen, birth weight, and gestational age are the major risk factors for the development of retinopathy of prematurity (ROP).
- Premature infants at or less than 1500 g or 30 weeks born in the United States should be screened for ROP.
- Current treatment of threshold or type I ROP is laser photocoagulation of the peripheral avascular retina.
- Vascular endothelial growth factor inhibitors such as bevacizumab are the newest treatment option, but more research into dosage, safety, and long-term outcomes must be performed.
- All former premature children are at risk for high refractive error, amblyopia, and strabismus.

INTRODUCTION

Retinopathy of prematurity (ROP) is a potentially blinding retinal vascular disease that occurs in very low birth weight (VLBW) (<1500 g) premature infants. Originally called retrolental fibroplasia (RLF), the disease was first described in 1942.[1] In 1950, RLF was responsible for 21.5% to 41.7% of all childhood blindness.[2] High supplemental oxygen and lower birth weight were discovered to be the major risk factors in RLF.[3] Nevertheless, even with monitoring oxygen saturations in the 1980s, 5% of infants with ROP became totally blind.[4] Screening for ROP, close monitoring of prethreshold disease, treatment of threshold disease with laser photoablation along with prevention of ROP and prematurity have become the foundations for preventing blindness.

EXTENT OF THE PROBLEM

According to the 2010 US census, the preterm birth rate (<37 weeks) was 11.99% of all births and the low birth weight rate (<2500 g) comprised 8.15% of all births.[5]

Department of Ophthalmology, Nationwide Children's Hospital, 555 South 18th Street, Suite 4C, Columbus, OH 43025, USA
E-mail address: cateolsonjordan@gmail.com

Pediatr Clin N Am 61 (2014) 567–577
http://dx.doi.org/10.1016/j.pcl.2014.03.003
0031-3955/14/$ – see front matter © 2014 Elsevier Inc. All rights reserved.

VLBW (<1500 g) birth rate was 1.45% and was unchanged compared with the previous year census. In 2008, 24% of VLBW infants died within the first year of life.[5] From 1997 to 2005, 0.17% of total newborns born in the United States had some form of ROP.[6] It is the third leading cause of childhood blindness in the United States (14%).[7] In highly developed countries such as the United States, only the smallest, youngest babies are likely to have ROP, because of improved control of risk factors and more aggressive management of unstable infants. By comparison, in Latin America and Eastern Europe, there are higher rates of severe ROP and blindness, and the disease occurs in older and larger infants compared with the United States.[8] In poorly developed nations, preterm infants do not survive long enough to develop ROP.[8] In 2010, it was estimated that globally 184,700 premature infants would develop ROP, and of those, 20,000 would become blind or severely visually impaired.[9]

CAUSE/CONTRIBUTORY OR RISK FACTORS

Risk factors:
- Birth weight[10–15]
- Gestational age[10–15]
- Poor weight gain[11,16]
- Low cortisol concentration[17]
- Dopamine-resistant hypotension[17]
- White race[10,13,14,18]
- Birth at an outlying hospital[13]
- Low insulinlike growth factor binding protein 3,[19] low insulin growth factor,[16,20,21] and low urine vascular endothelial growth factor (VEGF)[22]
- Hyperglycemia[12,16]
- Insulin treatment[16]
- Corticosteroid treatment[12,16,23]
- Insufficient intake of docosahexaenoic acid[16]

Associated conditions:
- Respiratory conditions such as bronchopulmonary dysplasia[6,12,15]
- Fetal hemorrhage[6]
- Intraventricular hemorrhage[6,12,15]
- Blood transfusion[6]
- Sepsis[12,15]
- Respiratory tract colonization with *Ureaplasma urealyticum*[24]
- Patent ductus arteriosis[12,15]

Protective conditions:
- Hypoxia[6]
- Necrotizing enterocolitis[6]
- Hemolytic disease[6]
- Breast milk[25]
- Improved nutrition (lipids and total calories)[26]
- Maternal preeclampsia[27]

SEQUELAE

Infants with regressed or treated ROP along with premature infants who never developed ROP should be appropriately referred to a pediatric ophthalmologist at a young age, preferably in the first 1 to 3 years of life, to evaluate for the following ophthalmic conditions related to both ROP and prematurity:

- Blindness[2,4,28]
- Retinal detachment[29]
- Cataracts[28,30]
- Glaucoma[31]
- High refractive errors,[28,32,33] including high myopia[34–37]
- Amblyopia[28,32,33]
- Anisometropia[37]
- Strabismus[28,32–34,38]
- Astigmatism[37]
- Nystagmus[34,39]
- Microphthalmos[34]
- Cortical visual impairment[39]
- Developmental, educational, and social challenges[40]

CLINICAL ASSESSMENT

Screening preterm infants for ROP should include those with birth weight of 1500 g or less or a gestational age of 30 weeks or less.[28] In addition, infants with a birth weight between 1500 g and 2000 g or gestational age greater than 30 weeks with an unstable clinical course may be examined if they are believed by the neonatologist or pediatrician to be at risk for ROP.[28] The initial examination is based on the infant's age. Infants born at 24 to 27 weeks postmenstrual age should start ROP screening examinations at 31 weeks postmenstrual age. Infants born after 27 weeks of age should be screened at 4 weeks after birth.[28]

Examinations can be performed in the hospital or as an outpatient. After pupillary dilation, an experienced ophthalmologist performs the examination with a lid speculum, scleral depressor, and binocular indirect ophthalmoscopy. Description of ROP depends on location, staging, extent, and presence of preplus or plus disease[41]:

- Location:
  - Zone I: radius of which subtends an angle of 30° and extends from the disk to twice the center of the macula
  - Zone II: edge of zone I to the nasal ora serrata and around to an area near the temporal equator
  - Zone III: the remaining temporal crescent anterior to zone II
- Staging:
  - Immature: before the development of ROP
  - Stage 1: demarcation line between vascular and avascular retina
  - Stage 2: ridge (line acquires width and height)
  - Stage 3: extraretinal fibrovascular proliferation (**Fig. 1**)
  - Stage 4:
    - 4a: extrafoveal retinal detachment
    - 4b: foveal retinal detachment
  - Stage 5: total retinal detachment
- Plus disease (see **Fig. 1**):
  - Increase in venous dilation and arteriolar tortuosity, poor pupillary dilation and vitreous haze
  - Present in at least 2 quadrants

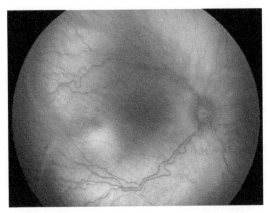

Fig. 1. Zone II, stage 3 with plus.

- Preplus: abnormal dilation and tortuosity of the posterior pole vessels (<2 quadrants)
- Aggressive posterior ROP (AP-ROP) (**Fig. 2**)
  - Most commonly in zone I but also in zone II
  - If left untreated, progresses to stage 5
  - Can be seen on the initial examination
- Regression of ROP[42]
  - Resolution without sequelae
  - Involution of the vasoproliferative phase to a fibrotic phase
  - Vascular abnormalities
  - Pigmentary changes
  - Temporal dragging of the macula
  - Traction and retinal detachment

Follow-up examinations depend on severity of the eye examination, with more severe examinations scheduled in 1 week or less and more stable examinations extended to 2 to 3 weeks. Examinations are terminated when retinal vascularization reaches zone III without previous zone I or zone II ROP, with full retinal vascularization

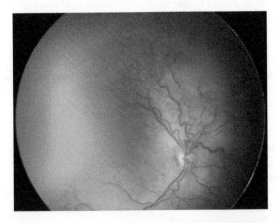

Fig. 2. AP-ROP.

within at least 1 disk diameter of the ora serrata, at postmenstrual age 50 weeks without previous prethreshold disease or with regression of ROP.[28]

In general, the screening examinations are safe and effective if performed by an experienced ophthalmologist. Even although these infants can decrease their heart rate and oxygen saturations in response to the screening examinations, there are not any clinically significant systemic complications directly attributable to ROP examinations.[43] These examinations can be made more comfortable by topical anesthetics,[28] pacifier sucking,[28,44] or sucrose.[28,45]

A carefully designed protocol to ensure appropriate screening and follow-up of infants at risk is a necessary component of ROP screening programs. Not only is there a grave risk of blindness when there is a delay in screening, referral, follow-up, diagnosis, or treatment, there is also a significant medicolegal risk to the physician and responsible hospital.[46,47] Evidence has shown that regional hospitals and higher-level neonatal intensive care units (NICUs) with such a protocol in place have fewer missed ROP examinations.[48] Maintaining a rigorous and safe ROP screening program is labor intensive. The increase in premature survival rates in developing countries, combined with the lack of fewer skilled ophthalmologists who can screen in moderately developed areas in Latin America and Asia, has led to an increasing incidence of ROP blindness.[8,49] New investigations into telemedicine screening to aid in these areas have shown promise. A recent study, telemedicine approaches to evaluating acute-phase ROP (E-ROP), had just been completed; however, results have not yet been published. Telemedicine involves training nonphysicians to take images with a retinal camera. The images are sent to an experienced ophthalmologist for interpretation.[49–51] There is evidence that telemedicine may be more cost-effective,[50,52] but binocular indirect ophthalmoscopy is the gold standard for screening ROP when there is an ophthalmologist to perform examinations. Recent studies might show that telemedicine is equally effective in diagnosing threshold disease, and this might become the standard in neonatal units that do not have a local pediatric ophthalmologist who can examine babies weekly. It is crucial that (1) all babies are tracked closely in the NICU, (2) babies are referred for immediate transfer if they have threshold disease requiring treatment, and (3) babies are referred for follow-up on discharge from the hospital. Ideally, the ophthalmologist reading the photographs should be the ophthalmologist who will follow the baby up for treatment if indicated. This practice helps expedite the process and decrease the chances for delay in transferring the infant to a center at which treatment can be performed.

MANAGEMENT

Historically, prevention of ROP focused on strict oxygen saturation guidelines. It is well known that high oxygenation increases the risk of severe ROP.[3,53] This situation is believed to be from oxygen-induced vascular closure and hypoxic stress, which increases VEGF.[54] Large studies have been conducted that have investigated target oxygen saturations. After collecting evidence from the SUPPORT,[55] Boost II,[56] COT,[57] STOP-ROP (Supplemental Therapeutic Oxygen for Prethreshold Retinopathy of Prematurity),[58] and HOPE-ROP (High Oxygen Percentage in Retinopathy of Prematurity)[59] trials, the safest target oxygen saturation for patient morbidity and mortality as well as reduction of ROP seems to be 90% to 95%.

The original treatment of threshold ROP was cryotherapy of the peripheral avascular retina. Threshold disease was defined as 5 contiguous or 8 cumulative clock hours of stage 3, in zone I or II with plus disease.[60] This treatment decreased unfavorable outcomes caused by ROP from 47.4% to 25.7%.[60] Subsequent investigations found that earlier treatment with laser photocoagulation had even better long-term results, with less initial pain and inflammation.[61]

Laser photocoagulation is now recommended for type I ROP (**Fig. 3**)[28,61]:

- Zone I any stage ROP with plus disease
- Zone I, stage 3 with or without plus disease
- Zone II, stage 2 or 3 with plus disease
- Treatment should be implemented within 72 hours of examination to reduce risk of retinal detachment

The newest treatment on the horizon is the off-label use of intravitreal VEGF inhibitors such as bevacizumab (Avastin). Bevacizumab is approved by the US Food and Drug Administration in colon cancer and has been used off label for treatment in adult macular degeneration and diabetic retinopathy. Intravitreal injections of bevacizumab have been used successfully for threshold ROP with half or quarter of the adult dose.[62–64] There are several advantages to using bevacizumab compared with laser, including:

- Rapid resolution of neovascularization and plus disease (**Fig. 4**)[62]
- Peripheral retinal vessels can continue to develop[62,63]
- Less invasive and does not require general anesthesia[63]
- Lower prevalence of myopia compared with laser after 1 year[63]

Disadvantages include:

- Peripheral retinal vessels take longer to mature, therefore requiring longer follow-up[62]
- Systemic absorption[63–65]
- Unknown dosage[63–65]
- Recurrence of ROP, requiring close observation after injection[66]
- Retinal detachment[54,66,67]
- Risk of infection (endophthalmitis), intraocular inflammation, increased intraocular pressure, ocular hemorrhage[68]

Intravitreal avastin should be considered only for zone I stage 3 with plus disease[28,62] and AP-ROP. Bevacizumab may also be used in conjunction with laser.[69]

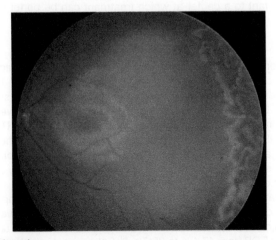

Fig. 3. Laser treatment.

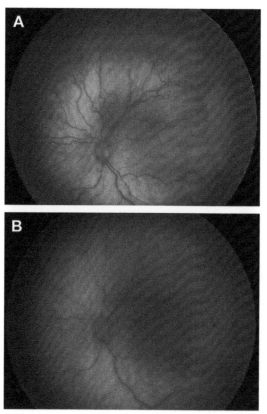

Fig. 4. (*A*) Zone 1, stage 3 plus, before bevacizumab injection. (*B*) Same eye, a few days after bevacizumab injection.

Because of the unknown long-term risks and need for close observation and longer follow-up, detailed informed consent for intravitreal bevacizumab must be discussed with parents.

SUMMARY

Extensive international experience along with large multicentered trials have established screening and treatment guidelines to prevent blindness or severe vision loss from ROP. New algorithms for screening and advanced treatments along with prevention of prematurity are the future of ROP management. Pediatricians should continue to be aware of the risk of high refractive error, amblyopia, and strabismus in all formerly premature infants, regardless of their history of ROP.[28,32]

REFERENCES

1. Terry TL. Fibroblastic overgrowth of persistent tunica vasculosa lentis in infants born prematurely: II. Report of cases–clinical aspects. Trans Am Ophthalmol Soc 1942;40:262–84.
2. Mallek H, Spohn P. Retrolental fibroplasia. Can Med Assoc J 1950;63(6):586–8.

3. Parmelee AH Jr, Pilger IS, Austin WO. Retrolental fibroplasia: a reduction in incidence following a decrease in use of oxygen therapy for premature infants. Calif Med 1956;84(6):424–6.

4. Ben-Sira I, Nissenkorn I, Grunwald E, et al. Treatment of acute retrolental fibroplasia by cryopexy. Br J Ophthalmol 1980;64(10):758–62.

5. Martin JA, Hamilton BE, Ventura SJ, et al. Births: final data for 2010. National Vital Statistics Report 61(1). Hyattsville (MD): National Center for Health Statistics; 2011.

6. Lad EM, Hernandez-Boussard T, Morton JM, et al. Incidence of retinopathy of prematurity in the United States: 1997 through 2005. Am J Ophthalmol 2009; 148(3):451–8.

7. Kong L, Fry M, Al-Samarraie M, et al. An update on progress and the changing epidemiology of causes of childhood blindness worldwide. J AAPOS 2012; 16(6):501–7.

8. Gilbert C, Fielder A, Gordillo L, et al. Characteristics of infants with severe retinopathy of prematurity in countries with low, moderate and high levels of development: implications for screening programs. Pediatrics 2005;115(5):e518–25.

9. Blencowe H, Lawn JE, Vazquez T, et al. Preterm-associated visual impairment and estimates of retinopathy of prematurity at regional and global levels for 2010. Pediatr Res 2013;74(Suppl 1):35–49.

10. Palmer EA, Flynn JT, Hardy RJ, et al. Incidence and early course of retinopathy of prematurity. The Cryotherapy for Retinopathy of Prematurity Cooperative Group. Ophthalmology 1991;98(11):1628–40.

11. Binenbaum G, Ying GS, Quinn GE, et al. The CHOP postnatal weight gain, birth weight and gestational age retinopathy of prematurity risk model. Arch Ophthalmol 2012;130(12):1560–5.

12. Mohamed S, Murray JC, Dagle JM, et al. Hyperglycemia as a risk factor for the development of retinopathy of prematurity. BMC Pediatr 2013;13(1):78.

13. Good WV, Hardy RJ, Dobson V, et al. The incidence and course of retinopathy of prematurity: findings from the early treatment for retinopathy of prematurity study. Pediatrics 2005;116(1):15–23.

14. Husain SM, Sinha AK, Bunce C, et al. Relationships between maternal ethnicity, gestational age, birth weight, weight gain and severe retinopathy of prematurity. J Pediatr 2013;163(1):67–72.

15. Tsui I, Ebani E, Rosenberg JB, et al. Patent ductus arteriosus and indomethacin treatment as independent risk factors for plus disease in retinopathy of prematurity. J Pediatr Ophthalmol Strabismus 2013;50(2):88–92.

16. Lundgren P, Stoltz Sjostrom E, Domellof M, et al. WINROP identifies severe retinopathy of prematurity at an early stage in a nation-based cohort of extremely preterm infants. PLoS One 2013;8(9):e73256.

17. Catenacci M, Miyagi S, Wickremasinghe AC, et al. Dopamine-resistant hypotension and severe retinopathy of prematurity. J Pediatr 2013;163(2):400–5.

18. Saunders RA, Donahue ML, Christmann LM, et al. Racial variation in retinopathy of prematurity. The Cryotherapy for Retinopathy of Prematurity Cooperative Group. Arch Ophthalmol 1997;115(5):604–8.

19. Gharehbaghi MM, Peirovifar A, Sadeghi K, et al. Insulin-like growth factor binding protein-3 in preterm infants with retinopathy of prematurity. Indian J Ophthalmol 2012;60(6):527–30.

20. Hellstrom A, Perruzzi C, Ju M, et al. Low IGF-1 suppresses VEGF-survival signaling in retinal endothelial cells: direct correlation with clinical retinopathy of prematurity. Proc Natl Acad Sci U S A 2001;98(10):5804–8.

21. Hellstrom A, Engstrom E, Hard AL, et al. Postnatal serum insulin-like growth factor I deficiency is associated with retinopathy of prematurity and other complications of premature birth. Pediatrics 2003;112(5):1016–20.
22. Levesque BM, Kallish LA, Winston AB, et al. Low urine vascular endothelial growth factor levels are associated with mechanical ventilation, bronchopulmonary dysplasia and retinopathy of prematurity. Neonatology 2013;104(1): 56–64.
23. Karna P, Muttineni J, Angell L, et al. Retinopathy of prematurity and risk factors: a prospective cohort study. BMC Pediatr 2005;5(1):18.
24. Ozdemir R, Sari FN, Tunay ZO, et al. The association between respiratory tract *Ureaplasma urealyticum* colonization and severe retinopathy of prematurity in preterm infants <1250 g. Eye (Lond) 2012;26(7):992–6.
25. Manzoni P, Stolfi I, Pedicino R, et al. Human milk feeding prevents retinopathy of prematurity (ROP) in preterm VLBW neonates. Early Hum Dev 2013;89(Suppl 1): S64–8.
26. VanderVeen DK, Martin CR, Mehendale R, et al. Early nutrition and weight gain in preterm newborns and the risk of retinopathy of prematurity. PLoS One 2013; 8(5):e64325.
27. Yu XD, Branch DW, Karumanchi SA, et al. Preeclampsia and retinopathy of prematurity in preterm births. Pediatrics 2012;130(1):e101–7.
28. Fierson WM, American Academy of Pediatrics Section on Ophthalmology, American Academy of Ophthalmology, American Association for Pediatric Ophthalmology and Strabismus, American Association of Certified Orthoptists. Screening examination of premature infants for retinopathy of prematurity. Pediatrics 2013;131(1):189–95.
29. Greven CM, Tasman W. Rhegmatogenous retinal detachment following cryotherapy in retinopathy of prematurity. Arch Ophthalmol 1989;107(7):1017–8.
30. Davitt BV, Christiansen SP, Hardy RJ, et al. Incidence of cataract development by 6 months' corrected age in the Early Treatment for Retinopathy of Prematurity study. J AAPOS 2013;17(1):49–53.
31. Bremer DL, Rogers DL, Good WV, et al. Glaucoma in the early treatment for retinopathy of prematurity (ETROP) study. J AAPOS 2012;16(5):449–52.
32. Cats BP, Tan KE. Prematures with and without regressed retinopathy of prematurity: comparison of long-term (6-10 years) ophthalmological morbidity. J Pediatr Ophthalmol Strabismus 1989;26(6):271–5.
33. Kushner BJ. Strabismus and amblyopia associated with regressed retinopathy of prematurity. Arch Ophthalmol 1982;100(2):256–61.
34. Gregory ID. Retinopathy of prematurity (retrolental fibroplasia) in children in whom the disease has not progressed to complete blindness, and the subsequent investigation of cases of myopia. Br J Ophthalmol 1957;41(6):321–37.
35. Nissenkorn I, Yassur Y, Mashkowski D, et al. Myopia in premature babies with and without retinopathy of prematurity. Br J Ophthalmol 1983;67(3):170–3.
36. Quinn GE, Dobson V, Davitt BV, et al. Progression of myopia and high myopia in the Early Treatment for Retinopathy of Prematurity Study: findings at 4 to 6 years of age. J AAPOS 2013;17(2):125–8.
37. Wang J, Ren X, Shen L, et al. Development of refractive error in individual children with regressed retinopathy of prematurity. Invest Ophthalmol Vis Sci 2013; 54(9):6018–24.
38. VanderVeen DK, Bremer DL, Fellows RR, et al. Prevalence and course of strabismus through age 6 years in participants of the Early Treatment for Retinopathy of Prematurity randomized trial. J AAPOS 2011;15(6):536–40.

39. Siatkowski RM, Good WV, Summers CG, et al. Clinical characteristics of children with severe visual impairment but favorable retinal structural outcomes from the Early Treatment for Retinopathy of Prematurity (ETROP) study. J AAPOS 2013; 17(2):129–34.

40. Msall ME, Phelps DL, Hardy RJ, et al. Educational and social competencies at 8 years in children with threshold retinopathy of prematurity in the CRYO-ROP multicenter study. Pediatrics 2004;113(4):790–9.

41. International Committee for the Classification of Retinopathy of Prematurity. The international classification of retinopathy of prematurity revisited. Arch Ophthalmol 2005;123(7):991–9.

42. The International Committee for the Classification of the Late Stages of Retinopathy of Prematurity. An international classification of retinopathy of prematurity. Arch Ophthalmol 1987;105(7):906–12.

43. Laws DE, Morton C, Weindling M, et al. Systemic effects of screening for retinopathy of prematurity. Br J Ophthalmol 1996;80(5):425–8.

44. Boyle EM, Freer Y, Khan-Orakzai Z, et al. Sucrose and nun-nutritive sucking for the relief of pain in screening for retinopathy of prematurity: a randomized controlled trial. Arch Dis Child Fetal Neonatal Ed 2006;91(3):F166–8.

45. Costa MC, Eckert GU, Fortes GB, et al. Oral glucose for pain relief during examination for retinopathy of prematurity: a masked randomized clinical trial. Clinics (Sao Paulo) 2013;68(2):199–204.

46. Demorest BH. Retinopathy of prematurity requires diligent follow-up care. Surv Ophthalmol 1996;41(2):175–8.

47. Bettman JW. The retinopathy of prematurity: medicolegal aspects. Surv Ophthalmol 1985;29(5):371–3.

48. Bain LC, Dudley RA, Gould JB, et al. Factors associated with failure to screen newborns for retinopathy of prematurity. J Pediatr 2012;161(5):819–23.

49. Skalet AH, Quinn GE, Ying GS, et al. Telemedicine screening for retinopathy of prematurity in developing countries using digital retinal images: a feasibility project. J AAPOS 2008;12(3):252–8.

50. Fijalkowski N, Zheng LL, Henderson MT, et al. Stanford University Network for Diagnosis of Retinopathy of Prematurity (SUNDROP): four years of screening with telemedicine. Curr Eye Res 2013;38(2):283–91.

51. Silva RA, Murakami Y, Jain A, et al. Stanford University Network for Diagnosis of Retinopathy of Prematurity (SUNDROP): 18-month experience with telemedicine screening. Graefes Arch Clin Exp Ophthalmol 2009;247(1): 129–36.

52. Jackson KM, Scott KE, Graff Zivin J, et al. Cost-utility analysis of telemedicine and ophthalmoscopy for retinopathy of prematurity management. Arch Ophthalmol 2008;126(4):493–9.

53. Cats BP, Tan KP. Retinopathy of prematurity: review of a four-year period. Br J Ophthalmol 1985;69:500–3.

54. Lee BJ, Kim JH, Heo H, et al. Delayed onset atypical vitreoretinal traction band formation after an intravitreal injection of bevacizumab in stage 3 retinopathy of prematurity. Eye (Lond) 2012;26(7):903–9.

55. SUPPORT Study Group for the Eunice Kennedy Shriver NICHD Neonatal Research Network. Target ranges of oxygen saturation in extremely preterm infants. N Engl J Med 2010;362(21):1959–69.

56. Boost II United Kingdom, Australia and New Zealand Collaborative Groups. Oxygen saturation and outcomes in preterm infants. N Engl J Med 2013;368(22): 2094–104.

57. Schmidt B, Whyte RK, Asztalos EV, et al. Effects of targeting higher vs. lower arterial oxygen saturations on death or disability in extremely preterm infants: a randomized clinical trial. JAMA 2013;309(20):2111–20.
58. The Stop-ROP Multicenter Study Group. Supplemental Therapeutic Oxygen for Prethreshold Retinopathy of Prematurity (STOP-ROP), a randomized, controlled trial. I: primary outcomes. Pediatrics 2000;105(2):295–310.
59. McGregor ML, Bremer DL, Cole C, et al. Retinopathy of prematurity outcome in infants with prethreshold retinopathy of prematurity and oxygen saturation >94% in room air: the high oxygen percentage in retinopathy of prematurity study. Pediatrics 2002;110(3):540–4.
60. Cryotherapy for Retinopathy of Prematurity Cooperative Group. Multicenter trial of cryotherapy for retinopathy of prematurity. One-year outcome–structure and function. Arch Ophthalmol 1990;108(10):1406–16.
61. Early Treatment for Retinopathy of Prematurity Cooperative Group. Revised indications for the treatment of retinopathy of prematurity. Results of the early treatment for retinopathy of prematurity randomized trial. Arch Ophthalmol 2003;121(12):1684–94.
62. Mintz-Hittner HA, Kennedy KA, Chuang AZ. Efficacy of intravitreal bevacizumab for stage 3+ retinopathy of prematurity. N Engl J Med 2011;364(7):603–15.
63. Harder BC, Schlichtenbrede FC, von Baltz S, et al. Intravitreal bevacizumab for retinopathy of prematurity: refractive error results. Am J Ophthalmol 2013;155(6):1119–24.
64. Harder BC, von Baltz S, Jonas JB, et al. Intravitreal low-dosage bevacizumab for retinopathy of prematurity. Acta Ophthalmol 2013. [Epub ahead of print].
65. Sato T, Wada K, Arahori H, et al. Serum concentrations of bevacizumab (avastin) and vascular endothelial growth factor in infants with retinopathy of prematurity. Am J Ophthalmol 2012;153(2):327–33.
66. Hu J, Blair MP, Shapiro MJ, et al. Reactivation of retinopathy of prematurity after bevacizumab injection. Arch Ophthalmol 2012;130(8):1000–6.
67. Jalali S, Balakrishnan D, Zeynalova Z, et al. Serious adverse events and visual outcomes of rescue therapy using adjunct bevacizumab to laser and surgery for retinopathy of prematurity: the Indian Twin Cities Retinopathy of Prematurity Screening database Report number 5. Arch Dis Child Fetal Neonatal Ed 2013;98(4):F327–33.
68. Falavarjani KG, Nguyen QD. Adverse events and complications associated with intravitreal injection of anti-VEGF agents: a review of literature. Eye (Lond) 2013;27(7):787–94.
69. Kim J, Kim SJ, Chang YS, et al. Combined intravitreal bevacizumab injection and zone I sparing laser photocoagulation in patients with zone I retinopathy of prematurity. Retina 2014;34(1):77–82.

A Review of Pediatric Idiopathic Intracranial Hypertension

David L. Rogers, MD

KEYWORDS

- Pediatric idiopathic intracranial hypertension • Pseudotumor cerebri • Papilledema

KEY POINTS

- Many children who suffer with headaches first present to their pediatrician for evaluation. Intracranial hypertension must be included in the differential diagnosis. Missing the diagnosis could result in permanent and severe visual loss.
- Idiopathic intracranial hypertension occurs in both children and adults.
- Making the diagnosis of idiopathic intracranial hypertension in a child can now be done with more confidence because of newly outlined diagnostic criteria.
- A significant percentage of pediatric patients with intracranial hypertension will have an identifiable secondary cause.
- Most children diagnosed with idiopathic intracranial hypertension will respond well to medical management alone.
- Surgical intervention is reserved for those who fail to respond medically.

INTRODUCTION

Idiopathic intracranial hypertension (IIH) is defined as elevated intracranial pressure (ICP) without clinical, radiologic, or laboratory evidence of a secondary cause. The most frequently cited incidence data for IIH in the general population of the United States are from a study by Durcan and colleagues,[1] who reported the incidence to be 1 in 100,000 individuals. When restricting the inclusion criteria to women aged 20 to 44 years, who are 20% or more above their ideal body weight, the annual incidence increases to 15 to 19 cases per 100,000 in the United States.[1] Although it has historically been described as a condition affecting obese women of childbearing age, it can occur in all age groups and genders in both obese and nonobese individuals and is becoming more recognized in the pediatric population.

Financial Conflict of Interest by Author: None.
Department of Ophthalmology, Nationwide Children's Hospital, The Ohio State University College of Medicine, 555 South 18th Street, Suite 4C, Columbus, OH 43205, USA
E-mail address: David.Rogers@nationwidechildrens.org

NOMENCLATURE

There has been much discussion and debate about the appropriate nomenclature to describe this condition. Historically, the condition has been referred to by terms such as meningitis serosa,[2] otitic hydrocephalus,[3] hypertensive meningeal hydrops,[4] pseudotumor cerebri,[5] benign intracranial hypertension,[6] idiopathic intracranial hypertension,[7] and, most recently, pseudotumor cerebri syndrome.[8] With so many names, confusion and misunderstanding can occur. The more descriptive term "intracranial hypertension," which is then further classified as either "idiopathic" or "secondary," is used in this discussion. The term "idiopathic" is reserved for those cases in which known secondary causes have been excluded. The term "secondary" is used for those cases in which an underlying cause is identified. These terms are simple, descriptive, and understood by all clinicians. It is important to recognize that little is known about the pathophysiology of IIH. It is quite possible that what is referred to today as "idiopathic" may likely become "secondary" as more is learned about the disease process.

DEMOGRAPHICS

More information is becoming available regarding the demographics of pediatric IIH. Current data suggest that prepubertal children affected with intracranial hypertension are more likely to be secondary rather than idiopathic in nature. In addition, the association with obesity and female gender does not hold true in this population.[9,10] Studies also suggest that IIH is infrequent in children less than 10 years of age[9] and extremely rare in infants less than 3 years old.

ASSOCIATED CONDITIONS

There are a myriad of secondary causes of intracranial hypertension and knowledge of these associated conditions will aid the clinician during the history and examination of the patient and can assist in guiding the subsequent workup. It is worth mentioning again that pediatric intracranial hypertension is more likely to be secondary in nature than idiopathic. Systemic conditions, cerebral venous abnormalities, drugs, endocrine abnormalities, and infectious causes have been identified as secondary causes of intracranial hypertension in the literature (**Box 1**). The exact mechanism by which these conditions result in secondary intracranial hypertension is not entirely understood in all cases.

CLINICAL PRESENTATION

The clinical presentation of pediatric IIH includes many of the same symptoms and objective findings as the adult patient. Headache is by far the most common symptom of IIH and occurs in more than 90% of cases.[11] There is no specific headache pattern that is pathognomonic of IIH; therefore, a thorough history and physical examination are needed to try and determine the need for further evaluation. Other symptoms include neck, shoulder, or arm pain, nausea, vomiting, pulsatile tinnitus, diplopia, blurred vision, and transient obscurations of vision.[12,13] Diplopia can be secondary to unilateral or bilateral sixth nerve palsies. The sixth cranial nerve is susceptible to damage from high ICP alone. Infrequently, patients may present with no suggestive symptoms at all and are only diagnosed when papilledema identified on routine eye examination prompts a further workup. For example, a thin 14-year-old girl presented for her regular eye examination and was found to have papilledema. She had been started on clindamycin for acne 8 weeks previously. Only retrospectively when prodded did she complain of new headaches. Within 2 weeks of stopping the clindamycin,

Box 1
Secondary causes and conditions associated with intracranial hypertension

Medical and Systemic Conditions	Infectious Diseases	Drugs
Head trauma	Bacterial and viral meningitis	Tetracycline
Subarachnoid hemorrhage	Lyme disease	Minocycline
Decreased CSF absorption from prior intracranial infection or hemorrhage	Human immunodeficiency virus	Doxycycline
		Nalidixic acid
Cerebral venous abnormalities	Poliomyelitis	Sulfa drugs
Bilateral jugular vein thrombosis or surgical ligation	Coxsackie B viral encephalitis	Vitamin A
	Guillain-Barre syndrome	
Increased right heart pressure	Infectious mononucleosis	Isotretinoin
Arteriovenous fistulas	Syphilis	All-trans-retinoic acid
Superior vena cava syndrome	Malaria	Amiodarone
Hypercoagulable states		Nitofurantoin
Renal failure		Lithium
Liver failure		Levonorgestrel
Sleep apnea		Growth hormone
Cystinosis		Thyroxine
Lupus		Leuprorelin acetate
Sarcoidosis		Steroid withdrawal
Hypoparathyroidism		
Addison disease		
Behcet disease		
Middle ear or mastoid infection		
Hypercapnia		
Pickwickian syndrome		
Anemia		
Turner syndrome		
Down syndrome		

all signs and symptoms resolved. Many children with refractive errors have experienced headaches when their glasses need updated, and it is possible for children to attribute blurry vision and headaches to the need for new glasses. This type of headache should be intermittent and mild.

EVALUATION

A thorough history is imperative when assessing a child with IIH. Both the parent and the child should be involved when the history is obtained, because the child's input can be a source of valuable information. The history should be focused on clarifying the patient's symptoms and identifying potential secondary causes. Demographic information should include the child's age, gender, and weight. Specific questioning should address stage of puberty, recent illnesses, medication use, recent weight gain, headache, nausea, vomiting, neck and back pain, systemic illnesses, and other neurologic complaints.

The clinical examination should focus on identifying features of IIH. Neurologic and ophthalmologic assessments are indicated. The ophthalmologic evaluation in the pediatrician's office should include a vision test, extraocular motility evaluation (specifically looking for abduction deficits that might indicate the presence of sixth nerve involvement), pupil evaluation, and examination of the optic nerve with a direct ophthalmoscope. The presence of disc edema in an undilated pupil can be very difficult to evaluate especially if it is very mild (**Fig. 1**). Moderate papilledema (**Fig. 2**) and florid papilledema (**Fig. 3**) are more obvious and can be accompanied by retinal hemorrhages and cotton wool spots. Pseudopapilledema can be caused by the presence of drusen buried in the nerve head (**Fig. 4**). Even if the nerves look normal (**Fig. 5**), this should not preclude referral to a pediatric ophthalmologist because the appearance might be evolving or disc edema could be absent. Evaluating the nerves and seeing any evidence of disc edema help the pediatrician make the referral emergent. The neurologic examination should be directed at identifying any focal neurologic deficits. If referral is warranted, the ophthalmic examination should be performed by an ophthalmologist familiar with the condition. The detailed examination should include assessing visual acuity, color vision, visual fields, extraocular movements, and a careful anatomic evaluation. Papilledema is the most important clinical finding because it is associated with vision loss, the most feared consequence of IIH. Photographs of the optic nerve are taken for monitoring purposes. The role of optical coherence tomography (OCT) in identifying and monitoring papilledema is not yet clear. The author currently performs this test on every patient and has found it to be a useful tool for monitoring response to treatment. OCT is a noninvasive imaging test that uses light to measure different layers in the retina and optic nerve. OCT is proven to be helpful in other ocular diseases, including glaucoma, diabetic retinopathy, and macular degeneration. If studies confirm that OCT is accurate and reliable in evaluating the response to treatment in patients with IIH, it will help decrease the number of lumbar punctures (LPs) performed on children with IIH.

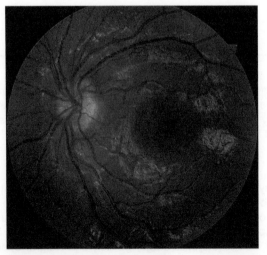

Fig. 1. Presence of disc edema in an undilated pupil.

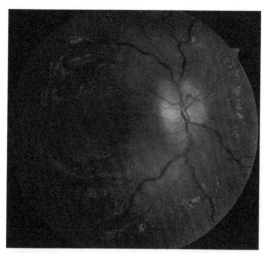

Fig. 2. Moderate papilledema.

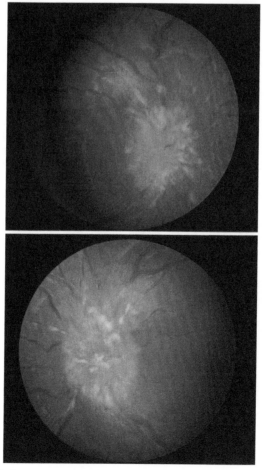

Fig. 3. Florid papilledema.

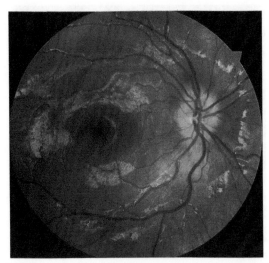

Fig. 4. Pseudopapilledema caused by the presence of drusen buried in the nerve head.

DIAGNOSTIC CRITERIA

Dandy[14] first presented diagnostic criteria for IIH without brain tumor in 1937. In adults, modified criteria are now used.[15] As previously mentioned, the pediatric patient with IIH is much different than the typical adult counterpart. Pediatricians and pediatric subspecialists familiar with these criteria frequently struggle to apply them in the pediatric population. The challenge of diagnosing pediatric IIH was recently addressed by Friedman and colleagues.[16] They proposed a modified criteria that include specific recommendations for determining if cerebrospinal fluid (CSF) opening pressure is elevated, one of the most difficult issues in the pediatric population (**Box 2**). These newly proposed criteria are comprehensive and also address an increasingly more common issue of diagnosing IIH in children without papilledema. Clinicians should be cautioned against empirically dismissing the diagnosis of IIH in pediatric

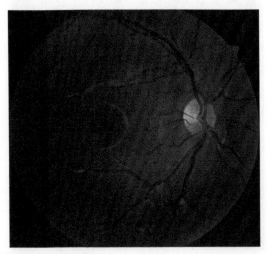

Fig. 5. Normal optic disc appearance.

approach for treating papilledema and alleviating symptoms.[35] Serial LP continues to be used to treat IIH. In some cases LPs are performed weekly or biweekly. In the author's experience, this is a poor treatment option because it has no long-term benefit, is painful for the child, worsens anxiety, is difficult in obese patients, and may require frequent sedation. LP is reserved for initial diagnostic purposes and subsequently only when needed to monitor CSF pressure in response to treatment.

SUMMARY

The diagnosis of IIH in a pediatric patient is becoming more common. The most important first step is including IIH in the differential diagnosis of any child with new-onset or chronic headaches. Understanding of the diagnosis and treatment of this condition has largely been based on data obtained in the adult population. Now a growing body of evidence demonstrates that pediatric IIH is quite different than the adult disease. An increased understanding of how this disease affects children has led to more specific diagnostic and treatment guidelines that will aid the clinician in treating these patients.

REFERENCES

1. Durcan F, Corbett J, Wall M. The incidence of pseudotumor cerebri: population studies in Iowa and Louisiana. Arch Neurol 1988;45:875–7.
2. Quincke H. Über Meningitis serosa: Sammlung linische Vortra 67. Inn Med 1893;23:655–94.
3. Symonds CP. Otitic hydrocephalus. Brain 1931;54:55–71.
4. Davidoff LM, Dyke CG. Hypertensive meningeal hydrops: a syndrome frequently following infection in the middle ear or elsewhere in the body. Am J Ophthalmol 1937;20:908–27.
5. Nonne M. Über Falle vom Symptomenkomplex "Tumor Cerebri" mit Ausgang in Heilun (Pseudotumor Cerebri): Über letal verlaufene Falle von "Pseudotumor Cerebri" mit Sektionsbefund. Dtsch Z Nervenheilkd 1904;27:169–216.
6. Foley J. Benign forms of intracranial hypertension: "toxic" and "otitic" hydrocephalus. Brain 1955;78:1–41.
7. Corbett JJ, Thompson HS. The rational management of idiopathic intracranial hypertension. Arch Neurol 1989;46:1049–51.
8. Johnston I, Owler B, Pickard J. The pseudotumor cerebri syndrome: pseudotumor cerebri, idiopathic intracranial hypertension, benign intracranial hypertension and related conditions. Cambridge (United Kingdom): Cambridge University Press; 2007. p. 1–356.
9. Babikian P, Corbett J, Bell W. Idiopathic intracranial hypertension in children: the Iowa experience. J Child Neurol 1994;9:144–9.
10. Scott IU, Siatkowski RM, Eneyni M, et al. Idiopathic intracranial hypertension in children and adolescents. Am J Ophthalmol 1997;124:253–5.
11. Wall M. The headache profile of idiopathic intracranial hypertension. Cephalalgia 1990;10:331–5.
12. Giuseffi V, Wall M, Siegel PZ, et al. Symptoms and disease associations in idiopathic intracranial hypertension (pseudotumor cerebri): a case-control study. Neurology 1991;41:239–44.
13. Binder DK, Horton JC, Lawton MT, et al. Idiopathic intracranial hypertension. Neurosurgery 2004;54:538–52.
14. Dandy WE. Intracranial pressure without brain tumor: diagnosis and treatment. Ann Surg 1937;106:492–513.

Box 2
Diagnostic criteria for IIH

1. Required for diagnosis of IIH
   A. Papilledema
   B. Normal neurologic examination except for cranial nerve abnormalities
   C. Neuroimaging: normal brain parenchyma without evidence of hydrocephalus, mass, or structural lesion and no abnormal meningeal enhancement on MRI, with and without gadolinium, for typical patients (female and obese), and MRI, with and without gadolinium, and magnetic resonance venography for others; if MRI is unavailable or contraindicated, contrast-enhanced CT may be used
   D. Normal CSF composition
   E. Elevated LPOP (≥250 mm CSF in adults and ≥280 mm CSF in children [250 mm CSF if the child is not sedated and not obese]) in a properly performed LP
2. Diagnosis of IIH without papilledema

In the absence of papilledema, a diagnosis of IIH can be made if B–E from above are satisfied, and in addition, the patient has a unilateral or bilateral abducens nerve palsy

In the absence of papilledema or sixth nerve palsy, a diagnosis of IIH can be suggested but not made if B–E from above are satisfied, and in addition, at least 3 of the following neuroimaging criteria are satisfied:
   i. Empty sella
   ii. Flattening of the posterior aspect of the globe
   iii. Distention of the perioptic subarachnoid space with or without a tortuous optic nerve
   iv. Transverse venous sinus stenosis

A diagnosis of IIH is definite if the patient fulfills criteria A–E.

The diagnosis is considered probable if criteria A–D are met but the measured CSF pressure is lower than specified for a definite diagnosis.

Adapted from Friedman DI, Liu GT, Digre KB. Revised diagnostic criteria for the pseudotumor cerebri syndrome in adults and children. Neurology 2013;81:1159–65.

patients without papilledema and should use the diagnostic category "probable IIH" proposed by Friedman and colleagues in these patients.

WORKUP

If intracranial hypertension is suspected, the subsequent workup should be done as soon as possible. Initial neuroimaging, usually with computed tomographic (CT) scan, should be performed and, if unremarkable, an LP with opening pressure should be performed. Further workup should be directed to rule out secondary causes and should be guided by the history and examination findings. Therefore, the workup of any individual patient is unique. The following is therefore offered as a guide and should not be considered a comprehensive assessment approach. When an initial workup suggests possible IIH, urgent neurologic and ophthalmologic evaluations are mandatory. Other testing to rule out secondary causes should be guided by the history and physical findings.

The LP can be difficult to obtain in a child who is awake. Many times this test must be performed under sedation. The preferred positioning is in the lateral decubitus position. Measuring the opening pressure should be done routinely. CSF should be removed and sent for appropriate diagnostic testing. In general, a basic cell count and cultures are done with the addition of other tests as directed by the clinical history and examination. The CSF composition should be normal.

Interpreting results of lumbar puncture opening pressure (LPOP) in the pediatric population is difficult because of the lack of any large-scale normative data. However, there is growing evidence in the literature that can guide the clinician in interpreting these results. Current evidence suggests that the upper limit of normal for LPOP in children between 1 and 18 years of age is 280 mm H_2O,[17–19] whereas neonates have a lower threshold set at 76 mm H_2O.[20] However, these studies have small sample sizes, and guidelines based on age alone are problematic. One of the problems this creates is dealing with the ends of the spectrum, such as the 18 year old with LPOP that is considered normal at 270 mm H_2O but would be abnormal if at 19 years of age. An LPOP greater than 280 mm H_2O is clearly abnormal with or without papilledema. The author also considers an LPOP of 250 mm H_2O as being abnormal if papilledema is present in conjunction with other clinical signs, and symptoms are consistent with IIH.

Neuroimaging is required before a diagnosis of IIH can be made. In some cases, the initial workup for IIH is done as soon as possible because of the acute onset of symptoms. In this setting, a CT scan is usually done before performing an LP to rule out intracranial pathologic abnormality. A normal CT scan of the brain is never adequate in making the diagnosis of IIH. Magnetic resonance imaging (MRI) of the brain with and without gadolinium and MR venography are the studies of choice to rule out known secondary causes.[21]

To make the diagnosis of IIH, neuroimaging should demonstrate normal brain parenchyma without evidence of hydrocephalus, mass, or structural lesion and no abnormal meningeal enhancement.[16] However, several abnormal MRI findings have been reported. Some of these include empty sella, partially empty sella/decreased pituitary height, flattened posterior glove/sclera, enlarged optic nerve sheath diameter, increased tortuosity of the optic nerve, enhancement of the optic nerve, intraocular protrusion of the optic nerve, and slitlike ventricles. Flattening of the posterior aspect of the globe, protrusion of the optic nerve into the intraocular space, and slitlike ventricles are highly specific for intracranial hypertension.[22–25]

TREATMENT

The best approach to managing IIH is with a multidisciplinary team that at minimum includes a neurologist and an ophthalmologist. Other specialists such as a hematologist, nutritionist, and endocrinologist can be called on as needed. A good working relationship among these specialists is essential. For simplicity, designating one specialist to manage all aspects of pharmacologic treatment will prevent confusion to the patient, parents, and other members of the medical team. The neurologist is the ideal individual for this task. The ophthalmologist works closely with the neurologist to guide treatment based on the ophthalmic findings, whereas the neurologist manages the medications and monitors for systemic side effects and other issues.

Randomized clinical trials are lacking in the pediatric population and the treatment of IIH is largely based on evidence obtained in the adult population. Lowering ICP is the mainstay of treatment with a purpose of preserving vision and controlling symptoms. However, identifying and directing treatment at the underlying cause cannot be overemphasized. In general, medical management is used first and surgical treatment is reserved for cases in which medical therapy fails to control ICP or if visual function is threatened.

Weight loss should not be neglected in patients who are overweight. One case ries showed that a weight reduction of 6% can result in a reversal of papilledem Another study of obese women with IIH showed that weight loss effectively redu not only headaches and papilledema, but also ICP.[27] Fortunately, most cases of diatric IIH will respond well to treatment; however, a small percentage will h some degree of permanent visual loss.[28–30]

EMERGENT TREATMENT

Initial treatment is aimed at lowering ICP and preserving visual function. In case where visual function is threatened because of severe papilledema, emergent neur surgical CSF diversion may be required. However, medical management should n be delayed. A short course of high-dose oral or intravenous steroids can be used addition to either oral or intravenous acetazolamide. The patient should be monitore clinically for signs of deterioration in visual function. Optic nerve sheath fenestratio (ONSF) is typically reserved for cases wherein acute elevation of ICP would threater visual function and to protect the optic nerve from further injury in recurrent cases. The ONSF should not be used as a long-term means of lowering ICP or as a treatment of headaches.

PHARMACOLOGIC TREATMENT

Carbonic anhydrase inhibitors have been shown to decrease ICP and treat papilledema.[31] Acetazolamide is the most commonly used carbonic anhydrase inhibitor. Furosemide is usually reserved for cases in which acetazolamide is not tolerated because of its minimal effect on lowering ICP. Topiramate is an antiepileptic drug with the secondary effect of inhibiting carbonic anhydrase. It has been used as an alternative to acetazolamide and has the added benefit of suppressing appetite, making it a good choice for those patients who are obese. The role of corticosteroids has not been proven; however, the author uses a short course of high-dose corticosteroids for acute cases of elevated ICP and papilledema associated with acute vision loss.

SURGICAL TREATMENT

The 2 surgical approaches used in the management of IIH are CSF shunting procedures and ONSF. In 1873, de Wecker[32] introduced the ONSF. It is used to treat papilledema that is unresponsive to medical management. Most patients have resolution of papilledema and stabilization of vision with this procedure.[33,34] From a vascular perspective, the optic nerve head is a delicate area described as a watershed. CSF pressure at the optic nerve head is thought to cause papilledema. The ONSF likely works by inducing a circumferential scar to form between the optic nerve sheath and the optic nerve directly behind the globe, effectively redirecting the pressure head of CSF from the optic nerve head and moving it posteriorly to an area that is more resilient. This theory is supported by the fact that ICP remains elevated after ONSF and that the fenestration itself scar down and does not remain open over time.[35–39] This simple explanation does not entirely explain the mechanism by which the ONSF works, as there are reports of patients who have had unilateral ONSF that resulted in a resolution of papilledema in the fellow eye and improvement in headache.[33,34,40,41]

There are several CSF shunting options but the 2 most frequently used approaches are lumboperitoneal shunt and ventriculoperitoneal shunt. It is the author's experience as well as the experience of others that lumboperitoneal shunting is the most effective

15. Digre KB, Corbett JJ. Idiopathic intracranial hypertension (pseudotumor cerebri): a reappraisal. Neurology 2001;7:2–67.
16. Friedman DI, Liu GT, Digre KB. Revised diagnostic criteria for the pseudotumor cerebri syndrome in adults and children. Neurology 2013;81:1159–65.
17. Avery RA, Shah SS, Licht DJ, et al. Reference range for cerebrospinal fluid opening pressure in children undergoing diagnostic lumbar puncture. N Engl J Med 2010;363:891–3.
18. Lee MW, Vedanarayanan VV. Cerebrospinal fluid opening pressure in children: experience in a controlled setting. Pediatr Neurol 2011;45(4):238–40.
19. Avery RA, Licht DJ, Shah SS, et al. CST opening pressure in children with optic nerve head edema. Neurology 2011;76(19):1658–61.
20. Kaiser AM, Whitelaw AG. Normal cerebrospinal fluid pressure in the newborn. Neuropediatrics 1986;17:100–2.
21. Said RR, Rosman NP. A negative cranial computed tomographic scan is not adequate to support a diagnosis of pseudotumor cerebri. J Child Neurol 2004;19:609–13.
22. Brodsky MC, Vaphiades M. Magnetic resonance imaging in pseudotumor cerebri. Ophthalmology 1998;105:1686–93.
23. Yuh WT, Zhu M, Taoka T, et al. MR imaging of pituitary morphology in idiopathic intracranial hypertension. J Magn Reson Imaging 2000;12:808–13.
24. Agid R, Farb RI, Willinsky RA, et al. Idiopathic intracranial hypertension: the validity of cross-sectional neuroimaging signs. Neuroradiology 2006;48:521–7.
25. Jinkins JR, Athale S, Xiong L, et al. MR of optic papilla protrusion in patients with high intracranial pressure. AJNR Am J Neuroradiol 1996;17:665–8.
26. Johnson LN, Krohel GB, Madsen RW, et al. The role of weight loss and acetazolamide in the treatment of idiopathic intracranial hypertension (pseudotumor cerebri). Ophthalmology 1998;105:2313–7.
27. Sinclair AJ, Burdon MA, Nightingale PG, et al. Low energy diet and intracranial pressure in women with idiopathic intracranial hypertension: prospective cohort study. BMJ 2010;341:c2701.
28. Cinciripini GS, Donahue S, Borchert MS. Idiopathic intracranial hypertension in prepubertal pediatric patients: characteristics, treatment, and outcome. Am J Ophthalmol 1999;127:178–82.
29. Phillips PH, Repka MX, Lambert SR. Pseudotumor cerebri in children. J AAPOS 1998;2:33–8.
30. Youroukos S, Psychou F, Fryssiras S, et al. Idiopathic intracranial hypertension in children. J Child Neurol 2000;15:453–7.
31. Rubin RC, Henderson ES, Ommaya AK, et al. The production of cerebrospinal fluid in man and its modification by acetazolamide. J Neurosurg 1966;25:430–6.
32. de Wecker L. On incision of the optic nerve in cases of neuroretinitis. Fourth International Ophthalmological Congress: August, 1872. London: Savill Edwards; 1873. p. 11–4.
33. Lee AG, Patrinely JR, Edmond JC. Optic nerve sheath decompression in pediatric pseudotumor cerebri. Ophthalmic Surg Lasers 1998;29:514–7.
34. Kelman SE, Heaps R, Wolf A, et al. Optic nerve decompression surgery improves visual function in patients with pseudotumor cerebri. Neurosurgery 1992;30:391–5.
35. Rekate HL, Wallace D. Lumboperitoneal shunts in children. Pediatr Neurosurg 2003;38:41–6.
36. Spoor TC, McHenry JG. Long-term effectiveness of optic nerve sheath decompression for pseudotumor cerebri. Arch Ophthalmol 1993;111:632–5.
37. Billson FA, Hudson RL. Surgical treatment of chronic papilledema in children. Br J Ophthalmol 1975;59:92–5.

38. Burde RM, Karp JS, Miller RN. Reversal of visual deficit with optic nerve decompression in long-standing pseudotumor cerebri. Am J Ophthalmol 1984;77: 770–1.
39. Kaye AH, Galbraith JE, King J. Intracranial pressure following optic nerve decompression for benign intracranial hypertension. J Neurosurg 1981;55:453–6.
40. Brourman ND, Spoor TC, Ramocki JM. Optic nerve sheath decompression for pseudotumor cerebri. Arch Ophthalmol 1988;106:1378–83.
41. Corbett JJ, Nerad JA, Tse DT, et al. Results of optic nerve sheath fenestration for pseudotumor cerebri: the lateral orbitotomy approach. Arch Ophthalmol 1988; 106:1391–7.

The Pediatric Red Eye

Melissa M. Wong, MD, William Anninger, MD*

KEYWORDS

- Conjunctivitis • Red eye • Uveitis • Contact lens • Corneal abrasion

KEY POINTS

- If you have a visceral reaction when a child presents to your office with a red eye, take heart, because ophthalmologists do not like the chief complaint of "red eye" any more than you do.
- The red eye differential is broad, and if you do not treat or refer it correctly, it may walk back into your office days later with a vision-threatening problem.
- Many of the common causes of red eye are benign, but there are some dangerous diseases that should be recognized and referred.
- A thorough history is critical. Key questions include the onset, duration, unilateral versus bilateral, exposure to sick contacts, painful or itchy, discharge, and vision change.
- Refer if there is a significant change in vision, or severe photophobia and discomfort.

ETIOLOGY AND CONTRIBUTORY OR RISK FACTORS

The red eye is complex because it is a nonspecific sign. A red eye may involve the conjunctiva; episclera; sclera; cornea; eyelid; nasolacrimal drainage system; or an internal ocular structure, such as the retina or uveal tract. The cause may be trauma, inflammation, infection, foreign body, or structural, and the cause may be localized to the eye or there may be an underlying systemic disorder.[1-3]

The important thing to remember is that conjunctivitis may lead to blindness. A single episode of severe conjunctivitis can cause corneal scarring that could affect vision, or lead to conjunctival changes that become a chronic degenerative problem.[1-4]

TOOLS TO EVALUATE THE RED EYE

The pediatrician has the essential tools readily available to assess a red eye and determine a treatment path, or make the decision to refer. An essential first step is to put on examining gloves to prevent an epidemic of viral conjunctivitis. Checking the vision should be done immediately, because when there is decreased vision, regardless of

The authors have no conflicts or financial disclosures.
Department of Ophthalmology, The Children's Hospital of Philadelphia, 34th and Civic Center Boulevard, Philadelphia, PA 19104, USA
* Corresponding author.
E-mail address: anninger@email.chop.edu

Pediatr Clin N Am 61 (2014) 591–606
http://dx.doi.org/10.1016/j.pcl.2014.03.011
0031-3955/14/$ – see front matter © 2014 Elsevier Inc. All rights reserved.

the other physical findings, it is imperative to refer. There might be posterior involvement of the retina or choroid that is causing the eye to be red from inflammation. A dilated examination is necessary to make the diagnosis.

A penlight or direct ophthalmoscope aids in assessing the pupils, looking for corneal clarity, and observing the pattern of redness on the conjunctiva and/or sclera. Intense redness at the limbus, referred to as ciliary flush, is often more concerning than mild general redness because it usually signifies problems on the cornea or inside the eye. The eyelids should be lifted and pulled back to get a view of the entire bulbar conjunctiva (the conjunctiva overlying the sclera) and the tarsal conjunctiva (the conjunctiva overlying the inside surfaces of the eyelids). Using a blue filter after instilling a drop of topical anesthetic followed by a drop of fluorescein-stained saline, it is easy to determine if there is a defect in the corneal surface epithelium. This can happen from trauma or from infections, such as pseudomonas and herpes. Motility should be evaluated also because an orbital process might cause limitation of movement and pain with movement.

Culture swabs need to be available if there is a large amount of discharge, especially if there is concern for gonorrhea or chlamydia. Cultures of the cornea need to be done at the slit lamp with special instruments. If there is a history of trauma and there is a chance the eye has been penetrated, a protective shield should be placed and the child sent to the emergency room.

HISTORY

The history is very important when trying to determine the cause of a red eye. The first question should be to ask if there has been any associated trauma. It is important to know so that you can be suspicious for a penetrating injury. Be aware, children are not always forthcoming with an accurate history if they think their actions will get them in trouble.

Next you should determine the onset and duration and whether it is unilateral or bilateral. It is helpful to know whether it started simultaneously in both eyes, or the onset of the second eye occurred after several days. This points to viral conjunctivitis.

It is important to check the vision, but you also need to ask if there have been vision changes. Sometimes the visual acuity can be normal, but there are qualitative changes, such as a visual field cut.

Next, one should explore for associated symptoms, such as photophobia, pain, itching, and swelling. It is important to ask about contact lens wear, and whether the contact is still in the eye. Knowing that the rest of the family also has conjunctivitis helps to reassure that the redness is viral, and observation is appropriate.

Red eyes can be associated with many systemic illnesses (discussed later) (**Box 1**). That is why a complete review of systems is necessary at times to uncover the cause of the red eye. Often the child presents with various symptoms before the onset of red eyes. The red eye often helps solve the diagnostic dilemma.

THE RED EYE CAUSES AND TREATMENTS

The causes of red eye can be grouped by etiology. The major categories include infectious (viral and bacterial), inflammatory, traumatic, structural, toxic and chemical, related to external disease, and foreign body including contact lenses.

Viral Conjunctivitis

One can spot a child with viral conjunctivitis in the waiting room; after rubbing their red, glassy eyes and runny nose, they happily touch every toy, magazine, and surface

---

Box 1
Systemic associations with red eye

History of bone marrow transplant and/or history of graft-versus-host disease

History of radiation therapy

Herpes simplex virus or varicella zoster virus infections

Juvenile idiopathic arthritis, Kawasaki syndrome, inflammatory bowel disease, systemic lupus erythematosus, Sjögren syndrome

Stevens-Johnson syndrome, toxic epidermal necrolysis

Malignancy (mucosa-associated lymphoid tissue, lymphoma, sebaceous cell carcinoma, squamous cell carcinoma)

Mucous membrane pemphigoid

Autoimmune connective tissue disease

Vitamin A deficiency

Rosacea

---

possible until they can be called into the office. Symptoms of tearing, discharge without significant purulence, redness, and conjunctival chemosis (boggy swelling of the conjunctiva) predominate. Commonly, one eye is initially involved and then the other eye follows several days later through autoinoculation of the virus. History often highlights systemic upper respiratory infection symptoms, and sick contacts. Physical examination may reveal a palpable lymphadenopathy (**Box 2, Fig. 1**).

Box 2
Viral conjunctivitis: treatment and when to refer

Treatment: Viral Conjunctivitis

Supportive care

Symptoms should decrease within the first week but may persist

Antibiotics do not hasten the resolution of a viral conjunctivitis

Cool compresses, artificial tears for comfort

No school or daycare for several days because it is highly contagious

In severe forms of infectious and/or inflammatory conjunctivitis, a low-dose topical steroid may be indicated

- Given the possible side effects, standard practice patterns recommend topical corticosteroid drops be prescribed and monitored by an ophthalmologist

When to Refer: Viral Conjunctivitis

No resolution of symptoms within a week

If vision is affected

Severe photophobia or pain

Organized inflammatory membranes in the cul de sac of the conjunctiva

- These can lead to symblepharon (fusing of the eyelid conjunctiva to the eyeball) and require management by ophthalmology

---

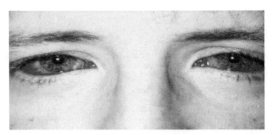

Fig. 1. Viral conjunctivitis. (*Courtesy of* Children's Hospital of Philadelphia, Philadelphia, PA.)

Pharyngoconjunctival fever

Pharyngoconjunctival fever is the most common viral conjunctivitis. It is associated with an upper respiratory tract infection and is typically caused by serotypes of adenovirus.[5–7]

A much more aggressive variant of pharyngoconjunctival fever is epidemic keratoconjunctivitis, which is more contagious and dramatic clinically. Epidemic keratoconjunctivitis is associated with a hemorrhagic conjunctivitis, and may lead to subepithelial inflammatory deposits of the cornea, which may blur vision and cause photophobia and pain (**Fig. 2**).[5–7]

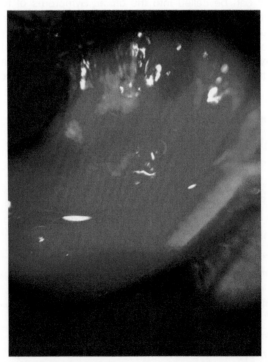

Fig. 2. Hemorrhagic conjunctivitis. (*Courtesy of* M. Wong, MD, Philadelphia, PA.)

Herpetic eye disease

Herpes simplex virus or varicella zoster virus can cause a conjunctivitis and severe eye damage. If there are vesicular lesions near the eyelid margin, eye redness in a patient with suspected zoster or herpes simplex, or a history of previous ocular herpetic disease, an urgent referral is warranted.[3,8]

Although varicella zoster tends to affect the thoracic dermatomes, the V1 distribution is a common area for the virus to reactivate. Herpetic corneal disease has a classic branching, dendritic pattern, best visualized with fluorescein staining.

Conjunctivitis associated with herpes simplex virus or varicella zoster virus should be evaluated by a pediatric ophthalmologist as soon as possible. Treatments include oral antivirals, such as acyclovir and valacyclovir, and topical antiviral and steroid medications. If the pediatrician is highly suspicious of herpetic eye disease, and immediate ophthalmology care is unavailable, starting oral acyclovir is appropriate (**Figs. 3** and **4**).

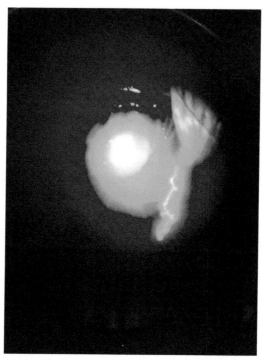

Fig. 3. Herpetic keratitis. A fluorescein stain reveals a linear staining pattern with branches, or dendrites, which are highly specific for a herpetic disease of the cornea. (*Courtesy of* M. Wong, MD, Philadelphia, PA.)

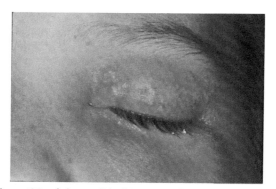

Fig. 4. Herpetic dermatitis of the eyelids. (*Courtesy of* Children's Hospital of Philadelphia, Philadelphia, PA.)

Molluscum contagiosum

Molluscum contagiosum is caused by a poxvirus and can lead to round, raised, flesh-colored bumps of the skin, with a small indentation. When near the eye, it can cause a follicular type of conjunctivitis that may be chronic. Given that each molluscum lesion releases virus particles, it can be difficult to eradicate with topical medications. The lesions may need to be frozen or excised to achieve resolution.[2,3]

Bacterial Conjunctivitis

The classic hallmark of bacterial conjunctivitis is unilateral purulent discharge. It is accompanied by redness and chemosis (swelling) of the conjunctiva. Bacterial conjunctivitis is commonly caused by normal flora of the body, such as *Staphylococcus aureus*, *Staphylococcus epidermidis*, *Streptococcus pneumococcus*, *Streptococcus viridans*, *Haemophilus influenza*, *Escherichia coli*, and *Pseudomonas aeruginosa*. Transmission is by direct hand-to-eye contact or from ascension from the patient's infected nasopharyngeal mucosa.

Acute bacterial conjunctivitis is of less than 3 week's duration. A careful history should be taken for febrile illness, other sick contacts, and concomitant genitourinary or gastrointestinal illness. As for all red eyes, vision and cornea checks are very important. Not all bacterial conjunctival infections are benign.

Neisseria-associated bacterial conjunctivitis is very purulent and has a severe onset of major symptoms in less than a day. Clinical signs of meningismus or significant febrile illness may indicate a conjunctivitis caused by bacteria, such as *Neisseria meningitides*; emergent referral to a hospital may prevent morbidity and mortality from meningitis. *Neisseria gonorrhea* and *Streptococcus pyogenes* are associated with corneal ulcer and perforation. Gonorrhea conjunctivitis may be associated with conjunctival membranes.

Chlamydia trachomatis is still the worldwide leading infectious cause of blindness, and may cause chronic follicular-type conjunctivitis with permanent scarring and inflammatory changes to the eye. Children with concern for gonorrheal or chlamydial eye infections should be referred to pediatric ophthalmology immediately.

Chlamydia and gonorrhea eye infections, when not in the neonatal period, may indicate sexual abuse. The clinician must be vigilant to explore this issue and if appropriate report to Child Protective Service, law enforcement, or public health institution as required by state or federal law.

Treatment

Topical antibiotic drops or ointment is the classic and effective treatment. Well-tolerated topical eye antibiotics include polymyxin B–trimethoprim drops, or erythromycin and bacitracin ophthalmic ointment. These are appropriate broad-spectrum first-line therapies. Good hand hygiene is very important, and patients and families should be educated. Flush with saline solution to remove purulence and decrease the bacterial load as needed.

A common question is whether or not to culture discharge. If there is marked purulence or a hyperacute onset of symptoms, then conjunctival culture is warranted. Also, culture should be performed in patients who are immunocompromised. If *N gonorrhea* or *C trachomatis* are suspected, a Gram stain and culture are indicated along with prompt referral to a pediatric ophthalmologist.

If a child is too uncooperative or uncomfortable to examine in the office, they should be referred to the ophthalmologist. The ophthalmologist can cheat and insert a speculum to get a better view. Clinical reasons to refer immediately include (1) decreased vision, (2) no significant improvement in symptoms within 2 to 3 days, and (3) evidence of corneal involvement.

Neonatal Conjunctivitis

Conjunctivitis occurring within the first month of life is termed neonatal conjunctivitis. Neonatal conjunctivitis may be a chemical or infectious conjunctivitis (**Fig. 5**).[2,9]

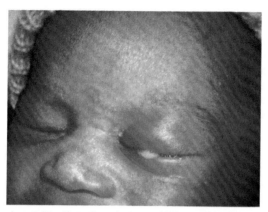

Fig. 5. Neonatal conjunctivitis. Note the relative puffiness of the left eye compared with the right eye, and the purulent drainage leaking out even with the eye closed. (*Courtesy of* M. Wong, MD, Philadelphia, PA.)

Chemical conjunctivitis has its onset within 24 hours of birth, and is a reaction to the topical bactericidal that was placed in the eye. Historically, silver nitrate or povidone iodine was used; antibiotic ointment, such as erythromycin, is common today. The symptoms resolve within days without a need for treatment.

Gonorrhea-associated conjunctivitis has an onset typically from 2 to 5 days of life, and is very purulent. This infection can be vision-threatening. Systemic treatment is with intramuscular ceftriaxone.[2,3,10]

Chlamydia-associated conjunctivitis typically occurs from 1 to 2 weeks following delivery. The discharge is less purulent then gonorrhea. Babies infected with chlamydia may develop pneumonitis. Treatment is with systemic and topical erythromycin.[2,3,11] In the setting of purulent neonatal conjunctivitis, consider empiric treatment of gonorrhea and chlamydia with intramuscular ceftriaxone and systemic erythromycin. Because gonorrhea and chlamydia may be coinfecting an individual, it is not unusual to treat empirically for both.

An infant presenting to your office with an aggressive conjunctivitis warrants emergent referral to a pediatric ophthalmologist, and may be admitted for systemic treatment and close monitoring for corneal involvement.

Eye examinations in neonates include checking for light aversion and a red reflex in each eye. If presenting with conjunctivitis Gram stain, Giemsa stain, and culture should be completed. A thorough review of maternal history is important. If gonorrhea or chlamydia is implicated, the infection was obtained via the birth canal, and the mother needs to be tested, treated, and counseled.

Viral conjunctivitis is rare in the neonate but can happen. If the history is suggestive, a viral conjunctivitis secondary to herpes simplex virus should be considered in unilateral conjunctivitis. Its typical onset is within 2 to 4 weeks of life. Treatment with a course of systemic acyclovir may be warranted because herpetic corneal disease can be vision-threatening. Any systemic signs of illness obviate a referral to the emergency room. In many cases, a herpetic infection of the eye may cause a limited blepharocon-junctivitis without vesicles and without corneal involvement, but then flare up when the child is older with corneal involvement.

Cellulitis

Infection of the periocular tissue presents as unilateral swelling, redness, and some-times tenderness of the eyelids. Often there is concomitant sinus disease with direct spread into the eye area, or a known scratch or bug bite. Urgent referral to ophthal-mology is warranted if there was trauma preceding the cellulitis, because it may be a reaction to a foreign body in the periorbital or orbital tissue.

Cellulitis occurs in two forms: preseptal and postseptal (orbital) cellulitis. The orbital septum is a connective tissue layer that acts as a theoretical barrier to infec-tious agents invading the deeper orbital tissues, the meninges, and cavernous sinus.[2,3]

Preseptal cellulitis presents with eyelid swelling and redness, a quiet white eye, normal vision, full motility, and reactive pupils. There is no pain with eye movement.

Postseptal cellulitis presents with eyelid swelling and redness, red or chemotic (swollen) conjunctiva, and possible decline in vision. There is usually limited motility or pain with eye movement and there may be a relative afferent pupillary defect. It might be subtle, and it is often difficult for the uncomfortable child to hold still and allow a detailed examination (**Fig. 6**).

Treatment of cellulitis

In children with preseptal cellulitis, it is reasonable to try a broad-spectrum systemic antibiotic, such as cephalexin (Keflex) or amoxicillin–clavulanate potassium (Aug-mentin). The patient should return for follow-up within 24 to 48 hours, and there should be a low threshold to refer if there is no improvement or orbital cellulitis is a concern.

Postseptal-orbital cellulitis requires admission and administration of intravenous an-tibiotics. Computed tomography imaging may be merited. Occasionally, surgical sinus or orbital drainage is required.

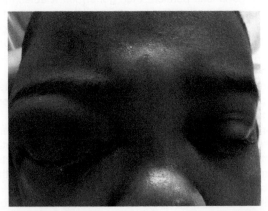

Fig. 6. Preseptal (periorbital) or Postseptal (orbital) cellulitis. (*Courtesy of* M. Wong, MD, Philadelphia, PA.)

Inflammatory Conjunctivitis

Allergic conjunctivitis may present with a similar appearance to viral or infectious conjunctivitis; however, the history is quite different.[2,3] The conjunctivitis should be bilateral, and itchiness and foreign body sensation are the predominant symptoms. There may also be redness and tearing. Refer to the article on allergic eye disease elsewhere in this issue for a full discussion.

Uveits

The uvea refers to the iris, the ciliary body, and the choroid, which are highly vascularized, pigmented intraocular tissues that may become inflamed. Uveitis may cause permanent vision loss and damage to all structures of the eye.

Children with uveitis may be completely asymptomatic, without redness, blurry vision, photophobia, or pain. This is why pediatric ophthalmologists screen many children on a regular schedule with such illnesses as juvenile idiopathic arthritis, which may predispose them to a silent uveitis.[2,3,12–14] If left untreated, silent uveitis can lead to cataracts, glaucoma, and other visually threatening ocular changes.

Some pediatric uveitis does present as a unilateral or bilateral red eye. If a red eye does not respond to initial treatments then a referral to ophthalmology is merited to check for uveitis. Uveitis may be caused by inflammation, infection, trauma, or neoplasm. The inflammation could be localized to just the eye or it could be systemic, such as arthritic involvement in juvenile idiopathic arthritis. Referral for any vague eye symptoms should be made in children with Sjögren syndrome, juvenile idiopathic arthritis, systemic lupus erythematosus, reactive arthritis, inflammatory bowel disease, nephritis, or granulomatosis with polyangitis.

Chalazion

A chalazion is the gift that keeps on giving. It is a collection of inflammatory debris in the oil glands of the upper or lower eyelid. It can present as a painless, firm subcutaneous nodule on the eyelid that waxes and wanes, seems to recur in different areas, and sometimes drains. Occasionally, it gets red, enlarged, and inflamed, and causes conjunctival reaction or even preseptal cellulitis. The chalazion is not an infection, and unless suprainfected does not respond to antibiotics (**Box 3**, **Fig. 7**).[2,3]

Box 3
Treatment: chalazion

They may spontaneously rupture and drain, or often diminish in size over months, with the assistance of daily warm compresses

Some children go through a phase of being prone to chalazia, and a regimen of eyelid hygiene may help keep them at bay (see **Box 4**)

Because they are inflammatory a limited course of topical steroid/antibiotic combination may help (eg, a combination tobramycin-dexamethasone drop or ointment)

If a chalazion has not decreased in size over several months with frequent warm compresses, then referral to an ophthalmologist for incision and curettage can be considered

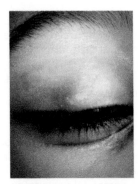

Fig. 7. Chalazion of right upper eyelid. (*Courtesy of* M. Wong, MD, Philadelphia, PA.)

Blepharitis

Blepharitis is a common cause of bilateral acute or chronic eye irritation. It can present as red eyes, and commonly has symptoms of chronic burning and itching. The issue is typically caused by a mixture of eyelid gland secretions and bacterial flora, most commonly *Staphylococcus* species.[2,3] Clinically, there are often small flakes and crusts at the eyelash-eyelid junction. There may also be chronic skin changes, such as eyelid thickening, redness, and scaling. Children with other skin conditions, such as eczema, often suffer with severe blepharitis (**Box 4**).

Box 4
Treatment: blepharitis

This is a chronic issue, and requires long-term and consistent treatment. First-line therapy is eyelid hygiene: careful scrubbing of the eyelash-eyelid margin with premedicated wipes or baby tear-free shampoo on a cotton-tipped swab or washcloth.

Like chalazia, benefit can be obtained from a short course of a topical antibiotic/steroid combination to treat the bacterial overload and knock back the inflammatory response. Common preparations include:

- Tobramycin-dexamethasone ophthalmic
- Neomycin/polymyxin B/dexamethasone ophthalmic

Lack of response merits referral.

Structural

The nasolacrimal duct system involves upper and lower eyelid puncta, which drain into the lacrimal sac and continue by way of the nasolacrimal duct, emptying into the inferior meatus of the nasal cavity.[2] Obstruction of the duct is common early in life, with a 95% spontaneous resolution rate by 1 year of age. Blockage can lead to a chronically wet, mildly irritated eye, and may lead to overgrowth of bacteria.

If there is focal mucoid or purulent material that can be expressed from the punctum, or a firm elevated nodule inferior to the medial canthus, the patient may have a dacryocele (cyst in the lacrimal system), or dacryocystitis, which is an infection within the lacrimal sac or cyst (**Box 5, Fig. 8**).

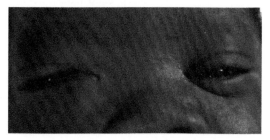

Fig. 8. Dacryocystocele or dacrocystitis. (*Courtesy of* M. Wong, MD, Philadelphia, PA.)

Fluorescein staining is important and often highlights a corneal foreign body or abrasion. A fluorescein dye examination is a very useful diagnostic tool because it highlights corneal and conjunctival defects (**Box 6, Figs. 9** and **10**).[2,3]

Be warned that proparacaine is a topical ophthalmic anesthetic and provides great relief. It is not to be prescribed. Overuse of the drop can cause damage to the corneal nerves, which predisposes to poor re-epithelialization and healing, and can lead to severe corneal damage. Patients occasionally steal the bottle seeking pain relief.

Box 6
Fluorescein technique

A topical anesthetic, such as proparacaine drop, is instilled in the affected eye.

Then a drop of the anesthetic is placed onto a fluorescein strip (sterile paper that is impregnated with fluorescein).

The strip is lightly touched to the inner aspect of the lower eyelid while the patient looks "up." Then have the patient blink.

Shining a cobalt blue filter light (which is a setting on most of the direct ophthalmoscopes) causes fluorescein to fluoresce green.

Dye staining in a pinpoint pattern or in a geographic pattern indicates a corneal or conjunctival defect, and may highlight a foreign body.

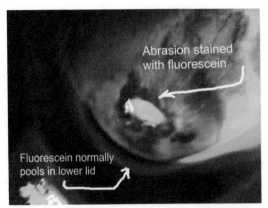

Fig. 9. Fluorescein examination. There is normal pooling in the lower eyelid, and fluorescein stains the tear film temporarily, which may spread unevenly across the ocular surface. Note that as the fluorescein dye dissipates and drains from the ocular surface there is a pooling and/or staining of dye in a geographic area, which indicates corneal abrasion. If the iris details are not visible because the cornea is whitened, then this is concerning for a corneal ulcer, which is an abrasion that has become secondarily infected or inflamed, and requires same-day evaluation by an ophthalmologist. (*Courtesy of* M. Wong, MD, Philadelphia, PA.)

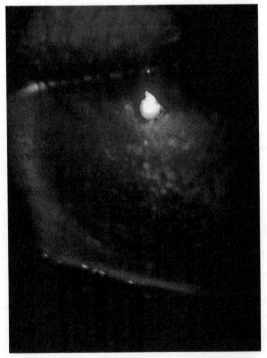

Fig. 10. Pinpoint fluorescein staining of the cornea, indicative of severe dry eye, which warrants treatment with artificial tears and lubricating ointment, or referral if severe. (*Courtesy of* M. Wong, MD, Philadelphia, PA.)

Trauma and Foreign Body

Corneal abrasion or foreign body

A red, irritated, or painful eye is often from a foreign body or corneal abrasion. The history may reveal a cause, such as a scratch to the eye, raking or playing in leaves, being at the beach, or hammering a nail. Close inspection of the eye may reveal the foreign body on the cornea or in the cul de sac of the eyelids. A corneal foreign body or abrasion can often be seen on red reflex with a direct ophthalmoscope. If a child suffers from a penetrating injury that involved a foreign body, it is important to ask for a detailed description of the "weapon" and examine it if you can to determine if there might be a foreign body inside the eye. A plain radiograph might be warranted if the object involved is radiopaque (**Box 7, Fig. 11**).

Box 7
Treatment: corneal abrasion and foreign body

For corneal abrasion initiate topical antibiotic treatment, and follow daily until resolution.

- Well-tolerated topical eye antibiotics include polymyxin B–trimethoprim drops, or erythromycin and bacitracin ointment. These are appropriate broad-spectrum first-line therapies.

- Second-line, more costly antibiotics include ciprofloxacin or moxifloxacin drops, which also have broad coverage.

If a foreign body is identified, irrigation with normal saline in a syringe or saline bullet often dislodges and washes it out.

Following successful identification and removal of the foreign body, topical ophthalmic antibiotic should be initiated with daily follow-up until resolution.

If you are not confident the foreign body has been removed, refer immediately to a pediatric ophthalmologist.

In the agitated child sedation may be required to remove a persistent corneal or conjunctival foreign body.

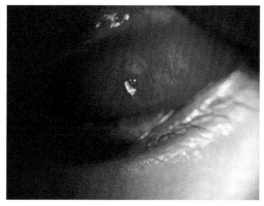

Fig. 11. Foreign body on everted eyelid. (*Courtesy of* M. Wong, MD, and G. Binenbaum, MD, Philadelphia, PA.)

Contact lens wear

A red, uncomfortable eye in a contact lens wearer merits immediate referral to the ophthalmologist. A contact lens is a foreign body and can be the origin of severe corneal infections or allergy-type reactions. Of particular concern is obtaining a history of sleeping without removing contact lenses. This can lead to ischemia of the corneal epithelium, and secondarily an infected ulcer. These ulcers can lead to permanent scarring and visual impairment. Contact lens overwear can also cause a chronic giant papillary conjunctivitis, which is essentially an allergy to the mechanical trauma of the lens. This contact lens intolerance can lead to an inability to wear contact lenses in the future.[3,15,16] Contact lens–associated ulcers can be very difficult to treat. There is no blood supply over the surface of the cornea; therefore, very frequent drops (sometimes every hour) are needed to treat the infection (**Box 8**).

Box 8
Treatment: contact lens

A contact lens wearer with a red eye, photophobia, or significant eye pain should immediately remove the lens and keep it out.

Complete a fluorescein dye examination in the affected eye as described previously.

For a simple abrasion topical antibiotic drops or ointment should be initiated immediately. Contact lens holiday until full resolution.

Have a very low threshold to refer this type of patient to an ophthalmologist.

Trauma

A red eye with a history of trauma merits immediate referral to an ophthalmologist, unless the vision is good, motility is normal, the cornea is clear, the iris is round, and there is a good red reflex.

Signs of a penetrating eye trauma include a peaked pupil, which appears like a tear drop; a disorganized anterior portion of the eye; prolapsing brown material; or visible blood in the eye (hyphema) and/or subconjunctival hemorrhage that is 360 degrees around the cornea or iris.[2]

If there is a concern for penetrating trauma by the history or the examination, the most important step is to put a shield (no eyepad) over the eye and arrange for an immediate ophthalmic examination or transfer to an emergency department. If no eye shield is available, a plastic foam or paper cup cut down makes an excellent temporary shield. Keep the child on nothing-by-mouth status in case a surgical repair is necessary.

Toxic and Chemical Exposure

When a patient presents to the office with a history of chemical or toxic exposure to an eye, the most important thing to do is irrigate the eye immediately. Do not refer to ophthalmology without initiating irrigation, unless the eye may have been involved in a penetrating trauma (do not irrigate this eye). Do not waste precious minutes to look up the pH and toxicities of every ingredient in the bottle of detergent or garage chemical.[3] Using tap water, or normal saline, copiously rinse the eye while trying to hold it open. Tilt the patient to the side, and rinse so the irrigant flows toward the ear and not toward the other eye.

Following irrigation, or if a patient's eye has already been rinsed, a pH paper strip can be placed into the lower fornix of the affected eye to assess that pH has been neutralized. It is best to check the pH a few minutes after rinsing so that the pH is not the pH of just the irrigating solution. Rinsing should be continued until the pH is normal. You can use an unaffected eye as a control if you are not convinced the pH is normal.

Following irrigation, or as a baseline examination, check vision and inspect the eye for redness of the conjunctiva and for clarity of the cornea. A fluorescein examination should be performed because many chemicals cause epithelial damage. If the cornea or conjunctiva has some staining, then follow corneal abrasion protocol, with follow-up in 48 hours to monitor for improvement. If the cornea shows any areas of whiteness, or you are concerned, the patient should be seen urgently by ophthalmology.

If one were to choose which type of substance would be thrown in an eye, acid would be preferable. Acidic substances cause denaturation of proteins, which prevents the substance from penetrating ocular tissues, whereas basic substances cause saponification reactions and allow chemicals to deeply penetrate ocular tissues.

REFERENCES

1. American Academy of Ophthalmology. Preferred practice pattern. Pediatric eye evaluations. 2012. Available at: http://one.aao.org/preferred-practice-pattern/pediatric-eye-evaluations-ppp–september-2012. Accessed February 18, 2014.
2. Basic and clinical science course 2013–2014, section 6: pediatric ophthalmology and strabismus. San Francisco (CA): American Academy of Ophthalmology; 2013–2014.
3. Basic and clinical science course 2013–2014, section 8: external disease and cornea. San Francisco (CA): American Academy of Ophthalmology; 2013–2014.
4. American Academy of Ophthalmology. Preferred practice pattern. Conjunctivitis. 2013. Available at: http://one.aao.org/preferred-practice-pattern/conjunctivitis-ppp–2013. Accessed February 18, 2014.
5. Wood SR, Sharp IR, Caul EO, et al. Rapid detection and serotyping of adenovirus by direct immunofluorescence. J Med Virol 1997;51:198–201.
6. Kinchington PR, Turse ST, Kowalski RP, et al. Use of polymerase chain amplification reaction for the detection of adenovirsues in ocular swab specimens. Invest Ophthalmol Vis Sci 1994;35:4126–34.
7. Shiuey Y, Ambati BK, Adamis AP, the Viral Conjunctivitis Study Group. A randomized, double-masked trial of topical ketorolac versus artificial tears for treatment of viral conjunctivitis. Ophthalmology 2000;107:1512–7.
8. The herpetic eye disease study group. Acyclovir for the prevention of recurrent herpes simplex virus eye disease. N Engl J Med 1998;339:300–6.
9. Conjunctivitis (Pink Eye) in Newborns. Centers for disease control and prevention web site. Updated January 9, 2014. Available at: http://www.cdc.gov/conjunctivitis/newborns.html. Accessed January 23, 2014.
10. Woods CR. Gonococcal infections in neonates and young children. Semin Pediatr Infect Dis 2005;16:258–70.
11. Darville T. Chlamydia trachomatis infections in neonates and young children. Semin Pediatr Infect Dis 2005;16:235–44.
12. Rosenberg KD, Feuer WJ, Davis JL. Ocular complications of pediatric uveitis. Ophthalmology 2004;111:2299–306.
13. Moorthy RS, Valluri S, Jampol LM. Drug-induced uveitis. Surv Ophthalmol 1998; 42:557–70.
14. Rolando M, Zierhut M. The ocular surface and tear film and their dysfunction in dry eye disease. Surv Ophthalmol 2001;45(Suppl 2):S203–10.

15. Dart JK, Radford CF, Minassian D, et al. Risk factors for microbial keratitis with contemporary contact lenses. Ophthalmology 2008;115:1647–54.
16. American Academy of Ophthalmology. Preferred practice pattern. Bacterial keratitis. 2013. Available at: http://one.aao.org/preferred-practice-pattern/bacterial-keratitis-ppp–2013. Accessed February 18, 2014.

Allergic Eye Disease

Virginia Miraldi Utz, MD[a,b,*], Aaron R. Kaufman, BA[c]

KEYWORDS

- Allergy • Conjunctivitis • Vernal • Atopic • Seasonal • Perennial

KEY POINTS

- Allergic eye disease is almost always bilateral, and itching is the predominant symptom.
- Allergic eye disease can be clinically and pathophysiologically classified as seasonal allergic conjunctivitis, perennial allergic conjunctivitis, vernal keratoconjunctivitis, atopic keratoconjunctivitis, contact blepharoconjunctivitis, and giant papillary conjunctivitis.
- The first step in management is avoidance of allergen and cessation of eye rubbing.
- For mild cases without evidence of corneal involvement, treatment with a combination of topical antihistamines mast cell stabilizers is highly effective, and topical nonsteroidal anti-inflammatory drugs and steroids should be prescribed by an ophthalmologist.
- The presence of pain, visual impairment, or evidence of corneal involvement should prompt referral to an ophthalmologist for further management.

INTRODUCTION

Ocular allergy, affecting approximately 10% to 20% of the US population, is one of the most common ocular disorders encountered by pediatricians and ophthalmologists.[1,2] Patients with ocular allergy often present with bilateral inflammation of the eyelid and conjunctiva that may be associated with rhinitis, asthma, or other atopic conditions. Allergic eye disease is classified into seasonal allergic conjunctivitis (SAC), perennial allergic conjunctivitis (PAC), vernal keratoconjunctivitis (VKC), atopic keratoconjunctivitis (AKC), contact blepharoconjunctivitis, and giant papillary conjunctivitis (**Table 1**). The predominant symptom is itching and redness, and mucinous discharge or photophobia may be present. If pain is present, vision is impaired, the cornea is involved, or symptoms do not improve with treatment, the clinician should refer the patient to an ophthalmologist. A basic understanding of eye surface anatomy is required to fully appreciate key diagnostic elements. Initial treatment involves a combination of topical antihistamines and mast cell stabilizers. Topical nonsteroidal anti-inflammatory drugs (NSAIDs) and occasionally short-term use of topical steroids should be prescribed ideally by an ophthalmologist, because

a Abrahamson Eye Institute, Cincinnati Children's Hospital Medical Center, Cincinnati, OH 45229, USA; b Department of Ophthalmology, University of Cincinnati, Cincinnati, OH 45229, USA; c Boston University School of Medicine, Boston, MA 02118, USA
* Corresponding author. Abrahamson Eye Institute, Cincinnati Children's Hospital Medical Center, Cincinnati, OH 45229.
E-mail address: Virginia.Utz@cchmc.org

Pediatr Clin N Am 61 (2014) 607–620
http://dx.doi.org/10.1016/j.pcl.2014.03.009
0031-3955/14/$ – see front matter © 2014 Elsevier Inc. All rights reserved.

Table 1
Clinical presentation and characteristics of ocular allergy

Characteristic	SAC	PAC	VKC	AKC	CBC	GPC
Age	All ages	All ages	<20 y (male>female)	Adulthood (male>female)	All ages	All ages
Onset	Childhood	Childhood	Preadolescence	Any age	Any age	Any age
Allergens	Tree pollens (early spring) Weed pollen (August–October) Outdoor molds Grasses (May–July)	Dust mites Animal dander Mold Air pollutants	Seasonal allergens	Any can contribute	Cosmetics Ophthalmic eye drops Inert chemicals	Foreign body Contact lenses Suture material Prosthesis
Seasonal	Yes	No	Yes	No	No	No
Personal or family history of atopy	Common	Common	Possible	Always	Possible	Possible
Contact lens wear	No	No	No	No	Possible	Yes
Symptoms	Itching Tearing Photophobia	Itching Tearing Photophobia	Itching Copious mucous Photophobia	Itching Burning Photophobia	Itching Burning Photophobia	Itching Tearing Photophobia
Pathophysiology	IgE-mediated Type I hypersensitivity	IgE-mediated Type I hypersensitivity	IgE-mediated Type I and IV hypersensitivity	IgE-mediated Type I and IV hypersensitivity	Type IV hypersensitivity	IgE-mediated Type I and IV hypersensitivity
Conjunctival eosinophilia	Yes	Yes	Always	Always (acute phase)	Occasional	Rare
Serum IgE	Mildly elevated	Mildly elevated	Elevated	Elevated	Variable	Variable
Goblet cells	Elevated	Elevated	Marked elevation	Decreased	Variable	Variable
Periocular skin involvement	Sometimes edema	Sometimes edema	Sometimes edema	Sometimes edema, sometimes eczema	Dermatitis, sometimes edema	Sometimes edema
Visual impairment	+/–	+/–	++	+++	+/–	+/–

Conjunctival reaction	Papillary	Papillary	Giant papillary reaction (upper tarsus)	Papillary reaction/thickened (upper tarsus)	Papillary or follicular response	Giant papillary reaction
Corneal involvement	+/−	+/−	++	++++	+	+
Skin tests	Positive	Positive	Positive	Positive	Variable	Variable
Natural history	Self-limited; symptomatic treatment	Self-limited; symptomatic treatment	Requires treatment; usually resolves by age 20 y	Chronic	Short-term; requires treatment	Chronic; contact lens associated
Concurrent ocular complications	None	None	Shield ulcer (sterile ulcer)	Cataracts Secondary infections (HSV, staphylococcal) Glaucoma	None	Peripheral corneal pannus
First-line prophylaxis	Avoidance Mast cell stabilizers	Avoidance Mast cell stabilizers	Mast cell stabilizers	Avoidance Mast cell stabilizers	Avoidance	Avoidance Mast cell stabilizers
First-line acute treatment	Topical antihistamine/mast cell stabilizers	Topical antihistamine/mast cell stabilizers	Should be treated by ophthalmologist Topical antihistamine/mast cell stabilizers Topical cyclosporine Topical mild steroid Allergist referral Possible systemic treatment Topical corticosteroid pulse	Should be treated by ophthalmologist Topical antihistamine/mast cell stabilizers Topical cyclosporine Topical mild steroid Allergist referral Possible systemic treatment May require chronic treatment Topical corticosteroid pulse	Mild topical corticosteroid to periocular skin	Topical antihistamine/mast cell stabilizers

Abbreviations: CBC, contact blepharoconjunctivitis; GPC, giant papillary conjunctivitis; HSV, herpes simplex virus; PAC, perennial allergic conjunctivitis; SAC, seasonal allergic conjunctivitis; VKC, vernal keratoconjunctivits; +/−, may or may not be present; +, sometimes present; ++, usually present; +++, often present; ++++, always present.

both medications can have complications that are difficult to recognize without a detailed ophthalmic examination.

CLASSIFICATION
Seasonal Allergic Conjunctivitis

Epidemiology and risk factors
Seasonal allergic conjunctivitis ("hay fever" conjunctivitis), representing 25% to 50% of cases of ocular allergy, is the most common allergic disease of the eye.[3] SAC is associated with hypersensitivity to airborne allergens, such as tree pollens (early spring), weed pollen (August through October), outside molds, grasses (May through July), or other environmental antigens depending on geographic distribution. Seasonal allergic conjunctivitis is most severe during the spring, summer, and early fall when the pollen levels are high.

Pathophysiology
Seasonal allergic conjunctivitis is classically a type I hypersensitivity reaction, caused by the binding of environmental airborne allergens such as pollen to IgE receptors in mast cells, which leads to degranulation of mast cells of the MC_T subtype. The release of proinflammatory mediators attracts eosinophils and basophils.

Clinical presentation
Seasonal allergic conjunctivitis is bilateral, with acute or subacute onset and peaks corresponding to seasonal variation in airborne antigens. Itching is the predominant symptom, although tearing, photophobia, and a burning sensation may be present. The eyelids and conjunctiva are typically involved. Conjunctival involvement may present as chemosis (swelling) and injection (redness), with chemosis more impressive than injection in most cases. Corneal involvement is rare, but mild punctate epithelial keratitis (small dry spots on cornea) may be present.

Perennial Allergic Conjunctivitis

Epidemiology and risk factors
Perennial allergic conjunctivitis has a similar clinical presentation to SAC, although usually milder. However, the allergens are often indoor antigens, such as dust mites, animal dander, and molds. Therefore, a definitive seasonal distribution is not uniformly present. The condition can be associated with dry eye syndrome, which is often undiagnosed in the pediatric population.[4]

Pathophysiology
Like SAC, PAC is IgE-mediated mast cell degranulation (MC_T) of proinflammatory mediators with recruitment of eosinophils.

Clinical presentation
Patients with PAC present with milder disease than those with SAC, and itching is the predominant symptom. Chemosis is often more impressive than conjunctival injection, but both tend to be present. A fine papillary reaction is present on the palpebral conjunctiva (**Fig. 1**). Dry eye syndrome may exacerbate the condition and requires separate treatment. Corneal involvement is rare in PAC alone and is usually only identified in cases of simultaneous PAC and dry eye syndrome.

Vernal Keratoconjunctivitis

Epidemiology and risk factors
Vernal keratoconjunctivitis represents 0.5% of allergic ocular disease.[5] Vernal keratoconjunctivitis affects mainly children and young adolescents ages 11 to 13 years, with

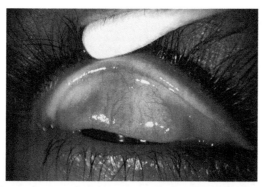

Fig. 1. Fine papillary reaction of the superior tarsal conjunctiva in PAC. (*Courtesy of* A. Kaufman, MD, Cincinnati, OH.)

a male predominance.[5] Both genetic and environmental factors likely play a role in the disease process. Approximately 50% of patients will have a history of atopy, such as asthma, allergic rhinitis, or eczema. Vernal keratoconjunctivitis is more common in hot and dry climates.

Pathophysiology

Although the precise pathophysiology is unknown, both type I and IV hypersensitivity reactions contribute to the pathogenesis,[6] with antigenic stimulation leading to lymphocyte (mainly T-helper type 2 [Th2] cells) activation with intense eosinophilic infiltrate. In addition, goblet cells are increased with elevation of mucin-5AC (MUC5AC) levels, and subsequent abundant mucous is observed with this condition.[7]

Clinical features

Bilateral, intense itching is the predominant symptom of this condition, often accompanied by photophobia and ropey discharge. Two anatomic forms exist: (1) palpebral, with giant upper tarsal papillae (>1 mm, often 7–8 mm), giving a "cobblestone" appearance on the surface of an everted eyelid (**Fig. 2**), and (2) limbal bulbar conjunctiva, which create gelatinous eosinophilic mounds (known as *Trantas dots*) at the limbus (**Fig. 3**). Both of these findings can be identified without ophthalmologic

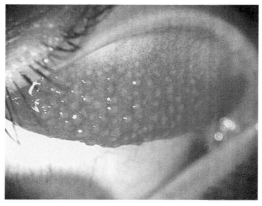

Fig. 2. Giant papillae of the superior palpebral conjunctiva in a patient with vernal conjunctivitis. (*Courtesy of* A. Kaufman, MD, Cincinnati, OH.)

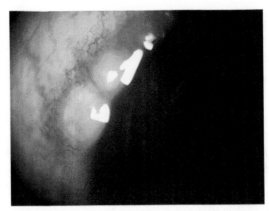

Fig. 3. Horner trantas dots in the limbal subtype of vernal conjunctivitis. (*Courtesy of* D. Saltarelli, OD, Cincinnati, OH.)

magnification. Eyelid edema is concurrent with conjunctival injection. Importantly, 5% of patients will have corneal involvement,[8] which can lead to visual impairment. If not treated, corneal involvement can eventually lead to permanent scarring. The giant papillae on the upper tarsal surface can cause mechanical trauma or "rubbing" of the cornea. A slit lamp examination is required to identify the following findings:

- Superficial punctate keratopathy: small pinpoint areas of fluorescein uptake on the upper half of the cornea
- Corneal macroerosions and/or shield ulcers: sterile infiltrate with overlying epithelial loss leading to intensely staining patch on the upper half of the cornea
- Superficial pannus formation and opacification of the cornea adjacent to the superior limbus

Decreased vision or suspicion for corneal involvement should prompt semiurgent referral to an ophthalmologist for further evaluation.

Atopic Keratoconjunctivitis

Epidemiology and risk factors
Atopic keratoconjunctivitis is a severe, chronic inflammatory disorder that is more common in adult patients aged 20 to 50 years, with a male predominance.[9] Some patients can prevent at a very young age. Personal and family histories are significant for atopic disease in 95% of patients, with atopic dermatitis the most common associated disorder.[10]

Pathophysiology
The immunopathology is complex, with both type I and IV hypersensitivity reactions contributing to the condition. Unlike with VKC, there is a reduction in MUC5AC-secreting goblet cells.

Clinical features
Symptoms of AKC include itching, burning, tearing, and erythematous/swollen eyelids. The eyelids have an eczematous appearance and there maybe madarosis (loss of eyelashes) from scratching. The chronic eyelid edema produces a classic Dennie-Morgan fold in the lower eyelid or an "allergic shiner."

Unlike VKC, the inferior tarsal conjunctiva is more likely to be involved with smaller (<1 mm) papillae. Chronic inflammation can lead to adhesions (symblepharon) within the lower fornix. Corneal complications are present in many patients with this disorder, and may include punctate epithelial keratitis (most prominent in the lower cornea), pannus formation, and frank ulceration. Patients with AKC have an increased susceptibility to herpetic keratitis, which can be severe and vision-threatening.

Contact Blepharoconjunctivitis

Epidemiology and risk factors
Contact blepharoconjunctivitis is secondary to re-exposure to cosmetics, chemicals, and some household plants (**Table 2**). Patients with and without atopy are affected.

Pathophysiology
Contact blepharoconjunctivitis is a type IV hypersensitivity response in which the allergen serves as a hapten (incomplete antigen) and combines with other proteins to form an immunologically active antigen. Langerhans cells, which are type 2 major histocompatibility complex antigen-presenting cells, present antigens to T-helper type 1 (Th1) cells in the regional lymph nodes. The sensitization phase develops over weeks to months, and the sensitized T cells migrate to the ocular surface and release cytokines and promote chemotaxis of other inflammatory cells. Unlike in SAC and PAC, in which inflammation occurs within 2 to 3 hours, the reaction to the offending agent takes 48 to 72 hours. This reaction should be differentiated from those to toxic or mechanically irritative substances, which manifest within 2 to 3 hours.

Clinical features
Contact blepharoconjunctivitis is characterized by symptoms of itching and burning. The conjunctiva is usually involved, and the eyelid has an acute eczematous,

Table 2
Common products associated with contact blepharoconjunctivitis

Class	Examples
Cosmetics	Nail varnish Eyeliner Mascara (often contain nickel) Soaps
Preservatives	Benzalkonium chloride (found in many topical ophthalmic solutions) Thimerosal (contact lens solutions)
Antimicrobial agents	Polymyxin Aminoglycosides Sulfonamides Trifluridine
Other ophthalmic medications	Atropine Homatropine Tropicamide Scopolamine Tetracaine Dorzolamide

erythematous appearance. The chronic phase leads to lichenification of the eyelid skin. The conjunctiva may have a papillary or follicular appearance. The lower cornea may demonstrate superficial punctate keratitis, usually in the lower half where the offending substance pools.

Giant Papillary Conjunctivitis

Epidemiology and risk factors
Giant papillary conjunctivitis most commonly presents in contact lens wearers. Patients with history of atopy are at higher risk, and materials such as contact lenses, ocular prostheses, suture material, or foreign bodies are often the inciting elements.

Pathophysiology
Mechanical trauma of the conjunctival epithelium stimulates a Th2 lymphocyte–mediated response. An allergic component may be involved when protein deposits on contact lenses or prostheses serving as allergens create a type I hypersensitivity response. Alternatively, protein deposits can serve as haptens and create a type IV hypersensitivity response in some cases.

Clinical features
The foreign body or contact lens may be present for months to years before symptoms occur. Symptoms consist of intense itching, mucous discharge, and photophobia. Giant papillae (>1 mm) are usually present on the tarsal surface adjacent to the foreign body. Removal of the foreign body, cessation of contact lens use, or change to other types of contact lens can alleviate symptoms.

CLINICAL ASSESSMENT
History

The history should include onset, duration, exacerbating factors, relieving factors, and previous episodes, with attention to seasonal variation. Current or prior treatments including duration and previous compliance should be evaluated. Personal or family history of atopy (asthma, eczema, or allergic rhinitis) should be evaluated. One should inquire about new pets, recent relocations, remodeling projects, or other household exposures. The predominant symptom is itching and the condition is usually bilateral (it can be asymmetric). Complaints of significant pain or blurring of vision unrelated to tearing should alert the clinician to alternative causes. The clinician should ask whether the patient had recent contact with anyone with conjunctivitis to rule out a possible infectious origin.

Examination

Examination should include evaluation of the body for other skin lesions (eczema) or mucous membrane involvement. The examination should also include palpation for preauricular or submandibular and cervical lymphadenopathy, because these findings would be more consistent with an infectious origin. Monocular best-corrected visual acuity (with the child in glasses if these are worn) should be measured with a near card or at a distance. Pupils should be examined for any evidence of afferent pupillary defect or asymmetry. Extraocular movements should be assessed. The eyelid skin should be examined and palpated. The upper and lower eyelid conjunctiva should be inspected for a papillary reaction or presence of a foreign body. Lastly, fluorescein should be placed in both eyes and examined under an appropriate blue light for any staining that would indicate corneal involvement (**Fig. 4**).

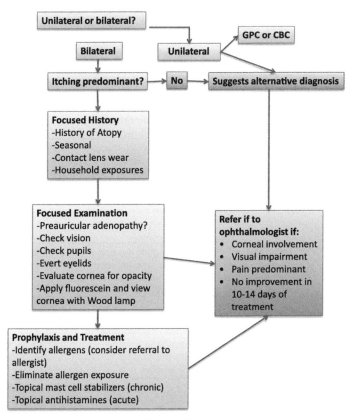

Fig. 4. Clinical evaluation and diagnostic algorithm for pediatric patients presenting with possible allergic conjunctivitis. CBC, contact blepharoconjunctivitis; GPC, giant papillary conjunctivitis.

Differential Diagnosis

The differential diagnosis includes infectious conjunctivitis, autoimmune origin (uveitis, scleritis), dry eye syndrome, and, rarely, congenital glaucoma. Distinguishing historical and examination findings are listed in **Table 3**.

MANAGEMENT

Avoidance of the offending antigen is the primary behavioral modification for all forms of allergic conjunctivitis. An allergist may be helpful in determining the specific allergens involved in severe cases by skin testing or radioallergosorbent test (RAST). Artificial tears can help to dilute the allergens and inflammatory agents and cool compresses may help in initial supportive management. When avoidance strategies and nonpharmacologic measures fail to control symptoms, over-the-counter (OTC) and prescription topical pharmacologic agents may be considered (**Table 4**). The mainstays of topical treatment by nonophthalmologists are largely antihistamines and mast cell stabilizers. In general, second-generation antihistamines are superior to that of first-generation antihistamines (see **Table 4**). Lodoxamide is more potent than cromoglycate in stabilizing mast cells and is faster acting [102]. Combination drugs

Table 3
Differential diagnosis of allergic conjunctivitis

	Examples	Historical	Examination
Infectious conjunctivitis	Viral conjunctivitis Bacterial conjunctivitis Fungal or parasitic conjunctivitis	Sick contacts Upper respiratory infection may accompany Eyes are involved sequentially rather than simultaneously	Preauricular lymphadenopathy Copious mucinous or green discharge
Autoimmune mechanism	Uveitis Scleritis	No itching May have systemic symptoms (joint/tendon pain) Ask about floaters Severe eye pain (scleritis) especially with ocular movements	May have decreased vision Systemic signs May be unilateral or bilateral
Dry eye syndrome	Aqueous tear deficiency Tear film instability	No itching (unless ocular allergy superimposed) Ask about medications that decrease tear production	Overlapping features with ocular allergy
Congenital glaucoma		Age <2 y Family history (usually autosomal recessive, so usually no history) Tearing Photophobia	Enlarged cornea Cloudy cornea (glossy appearance) Corneal asymmetry

such as olopatadine, ketotifen, and epinastine are efficacious in controlling both acute symptoms (H1 action) and prophylaxis (mast cell stabilization), and also increase adherence because of reduced dosing frequency. Topical decongestants should be avoided (oxymetazoline, naphazoline, tetrahydrozoline, phenylephrine). Although they cause vasoconstriction and can reduce erythema initially, rebound hyperemia and contact blepharoconjunctivitis can occur with acute and prolonged use respectively.[26] In general, topical NSAIDs and immunosuppressive agents (steroids, tacrolimus) should be prescribed by an ophthalmologist.

In terms of systemic treatment, first-generation antihistamines are not recommended because of their sedative affects and anticholinergic activity. However, second-generation antihistamines are widely used for allergic rhinoconjunctivitis and can be prescribed if systemic symptoms warrant. Importantly, systemic second-generation antihistamines can cause aqueous tear deficiency and dry eye symptoms that may actually exacerbate the ocular symptoms.[27]

SEQUELAE OF THE PROBLEM

Resolution depends on avoidance of allergen and/or compliance with appropriate treatment. The most serious sequelae are corneal involvement that can lead to scarring and visual acuity impairment. With the breakdown of epithelium with corneal involvement, the patient has increased susceptibility to bacterial or viral infections of the cornea. Evidence of corneal involvement or impaired vision should prompt referral to an ophthalmologist.

Table 4
Topical medications for allergic conjunctivitis

Drug Class	Example Medications Within Drug Class	Mechanism	Indications / Limitations/Complications	Selected Agents Dosing Requirements
Topical antihistamines	First generation: Antazoline, Pheniramine; Second generation: Levocabastine, Emedastine	Competitively and reversibly bind histamine receptors; No effect on proinflammatory mediators (PGs, LTs)	Acute treatment; Compliance (high dosing frequency with limited duration of action)	Levocabastine, 1 drop q6h ($\geq$12 y); Emedastine, 1 drop q6h ($\geq$3 y)
Mast cell stabilizers	Cromoglycate, Lodoxamide	Decrease in degranulation of mast cells, which prevents release of histamine and other chemotactic factors	Prophylaxis (requires a loading period 2–3 wk before antigen exposure); Compliance (high dosing frequency and need for loading period before symptoms improve)	Cromoglycate, 1 drop q6h ($\geq$2 y); Lodoxamide, 1 drop q6h ($\geq$2 y); Start 2–3 wk before allergen exposure[a]
Multimodal allergic agents	Olopatadine[b]	Selective H1 antagonist; Mast cell stabilizer	Acute treatment; Prophylaxis; Lower frequency of dosing	Olopatadine, 1 drop q12h ($\geq$3 y)[b]; Ketotifen, 1 drop q8h ($\geq$3 y); Azelastine, 1 drop q12h ($\geq$3 y) (less relief of itching); Nedocromil, 1 drop q12h ($\geq$3 y) (uncomfortable to instill, less effective than ketotifen and olopatadine); Epinastine, 1 drop q12h ($\geq$3 y)
	Ketotifen	Selective H1 antagonist; Mast cell stabilizer; Inhibits eosinophil activation, generation of LT and cytokine release		
	Azelastine	Selective H1 antagonist; Inhibits PAF; Blocks ICAM-1 expression		
	Nedocromil	Selective H1 antagonist; Mast cell stabilizer; Inhibits eosinophils		
	Epinastine	H1 and H2 antagonist; Mast cell stabilizer; Inhibits cytokine activation		

(continued on next page)

**Table 4
(continued)**

Drug Class	Example Medications Within Drug Class	Mechanism	Indications	Selected Agents Dosing Requirements
			Limitations/Complications	
NSAIDs[a]	Ketorolac Diclofenac Flurbiprofen	Reduce expression of PG D2 and PG E2	Additive drug to reduce hyperemia and pruritus Compliance: frequent dosing Complications: Asthmatic crisis[11] Corneal compromise[12]	Ketorolac, 1 drop q6h (≥12 y)
Topical steroids[a]	Fluorometholone Dexamethasone Prednisolone Clobetasone Rimexolone Loteprednol	Immunosuppressive and antiproliferative properties	Short course of treatment Long-term use for severe disease	Rimexolone, 1 drop q6h (≥12 y) Loteprednol, 1 drop q6h (≥3 y)

Topical medications are not approved for children ≤2 years of age.
Highlighted medications are author's favorite based on literature review.[13–25]
Abbreviations: H1, histamine type 1 receptor; H2, histamine type 2 receptor; ICAM-1, intracellular adhesion molecular 1; LT, leukotrienes; NSAIDs, nonsteroidal anti-inflammatory medications; PAF, platelet activating factor; PG, prostaglandin.
[a] Agents should be prescribed by an ophthalmologist for more serious disease.
[b] Formulation with once-daily dosing available.

ACKNOWLEDGMENTS

Special thanks to Adam H. Kaufman, MD, for reviewing this article and providing clinical images. Special thanks to Daniele Saltarelli, OD, for providing clinical images.

REFERENCES

1. Singh K, Axelrod S, Bielory L. The epidemiology of ocular and nasal allergy in the United States, 1988-1994. J Allergy Clin Immunol 2010;126(4):778–83.e6.
2. Bremond-Gignac D. The clinical spectrum of ocular allergy. Curr Allergy Asthma Rep 2002;2(4):321–4.
3. Chigbu DI. The pathophysiology of ocular allergy: a review. Cont Lens Anterior Eye 2009;32(1):3–15 [quiz: 43–4].
4. Kari O, Saari KM. Diagnostics and new developments in the treatment of ocular allergies. Curr Allergy Asthma Rep 2012;12(3):232–9.
5. Lambiase A, Minchiotti S, Leonardi A, et al. Prospective, multicenter demographic and epidemiological study on vernal keratoconjunctivitis: a glimpse of ocular surface in Italian population. Ophthalmic Epidemiol 2009;16(1): 38–41.
6. Hodges MG, Keane-Myers AM. Classification of ocular allergy. Curr Opin Allergy Clin Immunol 2007;7(5):424–8.
7. Hu Y, Matsumoto Y, Dogru M, et al. The differences of tear function and ocular surface findings in patients with atopic keratoconjunctivitis and vernal keratoconjunctivitis. Allergy 2007;62(8):917–25.
8. Bonini S, Coassin M, Aronni S, et al. Vernal keratoconjunctivitis. Eye (Lond) 2004; 18(4):345–51.
9. Bonini S. Atopic keratoconjunctivitis. Allergy 2004;59(Suppl 78):71–3.
10. Foster CS, Calonge M. Atopic keratoconjunctivitis. Ophthalmology 1990;97(8): 992–1000.
11. Sitenga GL, Ing EB, Van Dellen RG, et al. Asthma caused by topical application of ketorolac. Ophthalmology 1996;103(6):890–2.
12. Flach AJ. Corneal melts associated with topically applied nonsteroidal anti-inflammatory drugs. Trans Am Ophthalmol Soc 2001;99:205–10 [discussion: 210–2].
13. Leonardi A, Zafirakis P. Efficacy and comfort of olopatadine versus ketotifen ophthalmic solutions: a double-masked, environmental study of patient preference. Curr Med Res Opin 2004;20(8):1167–73.
14. Lanier BQ, Finegold I, D'Arienzo P, et al. Clinical efficacy of olopatadine vs epinastine ophthalmic solution in the conjunctival allergen challenge model. Curr Med Res Opin 2004;20(8):1227–33.
15. Lanier BQ, Gross RD, Marks BB, et al. Olopatadine ophthalmic solution adjunctive to loratadine compared with loratadine alone in patients with active seasonal allergic conjunctivitis symptoms. Ann Allergy Asthma Immunol 2001;86(6):641–8.
16. Abelson MB, George MA, Schaefer K, et al. Evaluation of the new ophthalmic antihistamine, 0.05% levocabastine, in the clinical allergen challenge model of allergic conjunctivitis. J Allergy Clin Immunol 1994;94(3 Pt 1):458–64.
17. Abelson MB, George MA, Smith LM. Evaluation of 0.05% levocabastine versus 4% sodium cromolyn in the allergen challenge model. Ophthalmology 1995; 102(2):310–6.
18. Abelson MB, Gomes PJ. Olopatadine 0.2% ophthalmic solution: the first ophthalmic antiallergy agent with once-daily dosing. Expert Opin Drug Metab Toxicol 2008;4(4):453–61.

19. Abelson MB, Greiner JV. Comparative efficacy of olopatadine 0.1% ophthalmic solution versus levocabastine 0.05% ophthalmic suspension using the conjunctival allergen challenge model. Curr Med Res Opin 2004;20(12):1953–8.

20. Abelson MB, Weintraub D. Levocabastine eye drops: a new approach for the treatment of acute allergic conjunctivitis. Eur J Ophthalmol 1994;4(2):91–101.

21. Abelson MB, Welch DL. An evaluation of onset and duration of action of patanol (olopatadine hydrochloride ophthalmic solution 0.1%) compared to Claritin (loratadine 10 mg) tablets in acute allergic conjunctivitis in the conjunctival allergen challenge model. Acta Ophthalmol Scand Suppl 2000;(230):60–3.

22. Borazan M, Karalezli A, Akova YA, et al. Efficacy of olopatadine HCl 0.1%, ketotifen fumarate 0.025%, epinastine HCl 0.05%, emedastine 0.05% and fluorometholone acetate 0.1% ophthalmic solutions for seasonal allergic conjunctivitis: a placebo-controlled environmental trial. Acta Ophthalmol 2009;87(5):549–54.

23. Deschenes J, Discepola M, Abelson M. Comparative evaluation of olopatadine ophthalmic solution (0.1%) versus ketorolac ophthalmic solution (0.5%) using the provocative antigen challenge model. Acta Ophthalmol Scand Suppl 1999;(228): 47–52.

24. Discepola M, Deschenes J, Abelson M. Comparison of the topical ocular antiallergic efficacy of emedastine 0.05% ophthalmic solution to ketorolac 0.5% ophthalmic solution in a clinical model of allergic conjunctivitis. Acta Ophthalmol Scand Suppl 1999;(228):43–6.

25. Fahy GT, Easty DL, Collum LM, et al. Randomised double-masked trial of lodoxamide and sodium cromoglycate in allergic eye disease. A multicentre study. Eur J Ophthalmol 1992;2(3):144–9.

26. Abelson MB, Paradis A, George MA, et al. Effects of Vasocon-A in the allergen challenge model of acute allergic conjunctivitis. Arch Ophthalmol 1990;108(4): 520–4.

27. Welch D, Ousler GW 3rd, Nally LA, et al. Ocular drying associated with oral antihistamines (loratadine) in the normal population-an evaluation of exaggerated dose effect. Adv Exp Med Biol 2002;506(Pt B):1051–5.

Convergence Insufficiency and Vision Therapy

Mary Lou McGregor, MD

KEYWORDS

- Vision therapy • Convergence insufficiency • Near point of convergence
- Home-based convergence therapy/In-office convergence therapy
- Dyslexia and learning disabilities

KEY POINTS

- Convergence insufficiency (CI) is common in the general population with an incidence of 2.5% to 13%.
- The symptoms of CI are extremely variable and can include eye strain, diplopia, headache, and tiredness when reading.
- There are 3 components to CI and include (1) decreased near point of convergence, (2) near point exophoria at least 4 prism diopters greater at near than distance, and (3) decreased fusional amplitudes at near fixation.
- Convergence therapy is a scientifically proven form of "vision therapy" that is effective in improving symptoms and alignment in children with CI. Learning disabilities are not caused by eye movement problems and vision therapy has no role in treating learning disabilities.
- Home-based convergence exercises should be the first line of treatment because it can be very successful in some patients, is convenient, and is much more cost-effective than in-office therapy. In-office treatment should be reserved for children who fail to improve with home-based therapy.

Convergence insufficiency (CI) is a common binocular disorder in which the eyes do not work well at near fixation. The incidence of CI in the general population has been estimated to be 2.5% to 13%.[1–3] The near point of convergence (NPC) is reduced, and the eyes drift out as a fixation target is moved closer. The NPC is the closest distance in which the eyes can maintain clear and equal focus on a near accommodative target. In general, it should be less than 6 to 7 cm in healthy children (children with refractive errors should be tested with their glasses on).

Ophthalmology Clinic, Nationwide Children's Hospital, OCC Suite 4C, 700 Children's Drive, Columbus, OH 43205, USA
E-mail address: mlkmcgregor@gmail.com

Pediatr Clin N Am 61 (2014) 621–630
http://dx.doi.org/10.1016/j.pcl.2014.03.010
pediatric.theclinics.com
0031-3955/14/$ – see front matter © 2014 Elsevier Inc. All rights reserved.

WHAT ARE THE SYMPTOMS OF CI?

These symptoms may occur in children with CI while performing near tasks (reading, working on a computer, using a cell phone, playing hand-held video games, making crafts, and so on)

- Headaches
- Eyestrain
- Double vision
- Blurred vision
- Loss of place while reading
- Excessive tiredness when reading
- Covering one eye
- Complaints of the words moving on the page
- Short attention span for reading
- Constantly adjusting the distance of the book, phone, and other objects, to see better

These symptoms can be aggravated by illness, tiredness, anxiety, and stress.

All of these symptoms can be caused by other ocular and nonocular problems.

Any child with these symptoms deserves a complete eye examination to rule out other eye diseases that could cause some of these symptoms, such as dry eyes, strabismus, refractive errors, optic neuritis, iritis, and other diseases. Children deserve therapy for symptomatic CI.

Double vision may not be present even with an obvious eye misalignment because a child can ignore a misaligned image if the deviation starts at a young enough age (approximately less than 6 years old) when the visual system is still maturing. Suppression is the term used to describe the ability to ignore a second image. It is an acquired neurologic rewiring of the visual cortex. There may be a moment when the eye deviates outward in a child with CI and some children will complain of blurry vision instead of double vision.

HOW TO TEST CONVERGENCE AND DIAGNOSE CI

The pediatrician can easily perform a simple check for NPC.

This simple check should be done when a child is getting ready to start kindergarten, or sooner if a parent notices any sign or symptom that might indicate a problem such as winking an eye or a drifting eye. The test requires an accommodative target (small letters or a detailed small picture attached to the end of a tongue depressor; **Fig. 1**). The target should be positioned an arms' length away at eye level and brought toward the child's face. Ideally the child should read the letters as the stick is coming closer.

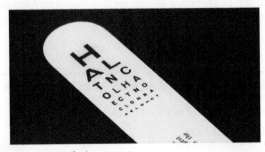

Fig. 1. Example of an accommodative target.

The tester should be observing the position of the eyes as they focus on the target. Accommodation is linked to convergence, and as the child focuses (accommodates), the eyes converge to stay focused on the same object. At some point the child will no longer be able to continue to converge and focus on the target. This point is referred to the near point of convergence (**Fig. 2**).

A pediatric ophthalmologist will perform 3 tests as part of the complete eye examination, before diagnosing CI. They include the following:

1. Cover test: This test is done to check for any misalignment of the eyes in the distance or at near. Other forms of strabismus can cause or aggravate convergence problems. If a child has an exotropia (manifest drifting out) in the distance, this can certainly affect the NPC. If the distance exotropia is poorly controlled or decompensates, surgery is often necessary. Once the distance deviation is taken care of, the near alignment can be evaluated. Often the near alignment is fine and no further treatment is needed. Some children have a CI type of exotropia whereby the near deviation is greater than the distance deviation. In these children, they often need surgery for the distance deviation and convergence therapy for the near deviation. In patients with CI, there is a near exophoria (latent deviation) of 4 or more prism diopters greater than the distance phoria.
2. Near point of convergence: This test should be performed several times as described above, looking for signs of fatigue. In patients with CI, NPC should measure greater than 6.
3. Convergence amplitudes: In this test a horizontal prism bar is held in front of one eye while the child tries to keep one of the target letters clear and single. The prism bar is slowly moved to increase the prism that the convergence effort must overcome. Eventually, the child cannot keep the image single and clear. This point determines the convergence amplitude (a measurement of the strength of convergence that often indicates the ability to maintain convergence without fatigue; **Fig. 3**).

SECONDARY CAUSES OF CONVERGENCE INSUFFICIENCY

1. Pseudotumor cerebri
2. Fourth nerve palsy
3. Duane syndrome
4. Traumatic brain injury/concussion
5. Behavioral medications
6. Distance exotropia

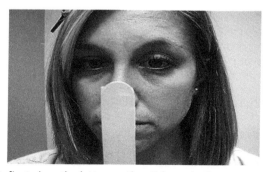

Fig. 2. A patient is fixated on the letters as the stick gradually moves toward the nose.

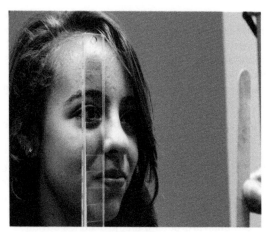

Fig. 3. Test to determine convergence amplitude.

After addressing the primary problem, these patients often need convergence therapy. With the new concussion guidelines recommending prolonged "brain rest" until symptoms resolve, it is important to consider that a prolonged headache associated with near work might be a symptom of CI and not unresolved brain trauma.

WHO NEEDS TREATMENT FOR CI?

There are 2 ways to approach CI. First, the convergence is evaluated and, if an abnormality is found, then the child or parent can be questioned about signs and symptoms. Second, screening questions can be asked to try and elicit signs or symptoms of CI, and then convergence can be tested if the child has any symptoms. The Convergence Insufficiency Symptom Survey (CISS)[4–6] was developed to help quantify symptoms before and after treatment of CI in children 9 years or older.

The questions of the CISS[4–6] include the following:

1. Do your eyes feel tired when reading or doing close work?
2. Do your eyes feel uncomfortable when reading or doing close work?
3. Do you have headaches when reading or doing close work?
4. Do you feel sleepy when reading or doing close work?
5. Do you lose concentration when reading or doing close work?
6. Do you have trouble remembering what you have read?
7. Do you have double vision when reading or doing close work?
8. Do you see the words move, jump, swim, or appear to float on the page when reading or doing close work?
9. Do you feel like you read slowly?
10. Do your eyes ever hurt when reading or doing close work?
11. Do your eyes ever feel sore when reading or doing close work?
12. Do you feel a "pulling" feeling around your eyes when reading or doing close work?
13. Do you notice the words blurring or coming in and out of focus when reading or doing close work?
14. Do you lose your place while reading or doing close work?
15. Do you have to reread the same line of words when reading?

In the Convergence Insufficiency Treatment Trial (CITT),[1] the patient answers each question with the following: never, infrequently, sometimes, fairly often, and always. There is an algorithm to calculate the score and this can be repeated after treatment to determine the subjective level of improvement and improvement in symptoms. These questions can give the pediatrician an idea of the types of questions to ask a child who has an apparent CI. These questions are very general and other problems can lead to positive answers. Comorbid ocular conditions can drive the results of the CISS. Referral is warranted for ocular symptoms that indicate the child is experiencing asthenopia or if there is an obvious reduced NPC. *Asthenopia* is the ophthalmic term that describes eyestrain or eye fatigue. Asthenopia (listed as visual discomfort) is a diagnosis with an ICD-9-CM code 368.13 and can be used by pediatricians when they see patients with any of the above complaints. The ICD-10-CM code is H53.143.

WHAT IS THE TREATMENT FOR CI?

Often a passive therapy is combined with various forms of an active therapy, especially when the child has accommodative deficiency or when the NPC is remote (**Box 1**).[7]

The CITT[1] was a prospective study performed in 9- to 17-year-old children. The goal was to compare the different treatments for CI. The study concluded that in-office convergence therapy (which was combined with home-based convergence therapy) was the most effective therapy in reducing symptoms and improving NPC and fusional vergences. The success rate was 73% compared with home-based pencil push-ups of 43%. The study looked at patients after 12 weeks of therapy. In a retrospective study completed by Serna and colleagues,[8] 92% of patients had a normalized NPC and improved positive fusional vergences, whereas 62% reported resolution of symptoms. Certainly there are drawbacks to retrospective, unmasked studies without controls, but the study does indicate that home-based therapy can be effective. Because of the high out-of-pocket cost of in-office therapy and the difficulty in adhering to a weekly schedule for busy families, it is reasonable to try home-based therapy as a first-treatment modality. Timing is not critical and, if children fail home-based therapy,

Box 1
Treatment options for CI

Passive therapy

1. Observation: Can be appropriate if the child is asymptomatic and the CI is mild.
2. Prism glasses: These may help with symptoms of diplopia but they do not provide effective treatment to improve CI.
3. Reading glasses: Often there is also an accommodative deficiency that is treated with prescription/over-the-counter reading glasses. Up to 78% of children with all 3 signs of CI also had accommodative insufficiency.[5]

Active therapy

4. Pencil push-ups done at home.
5. Home-based computer vergence/accommodative therapy with pencil push-ups.
6. Office-based vergence/accommodative therapy with home reinforcement.
7. Other orthoptic and binocular activities to stimulate fusion.
8. Surgery: Rarely recommended because of the high risk of double vision in the distance.

they can conceivably undergo in-office therapy. Compliance with the treatment regimen is critical for any convergence therapy to be effective.

CONTROVERSIES OVER VISION THERAPY BETWEEN THE OPTOMETRIC AND OPHTHALMIC COMMUNITIES

In 2009, Cacho Martínez and colleagues[9] published a review of the scientific literature to analyze the nonsurgical treatment available for accommodative and nonstrabismic binocular dysfunctions. The authors did an exhaustive search of the literature and determined that there is scientific evidence to support the claim that vision therapy (specifically a combination of active convergence therapy) improves symptoms and signs of CI only. They also stated, "For the other nonstrabismic binocular conditions and accommodative disorders, there is a lack of published randomized, clinical trials that support the evidence for the efficacy of each treatment." Although there are many published claims in the literature to support vision therapy for the treatment of a range of problems, unfortunately, there is no scientific data to support the claims.

The biggest controversy regarding the role of vision therapy is whether it helps with reading problems. The claim that vision therapy can improve reading skills in patients with abnormal saccadic movements is based on the theory that changes in the eye movements following saccadic vision therapy result in improvement of reading assessments. Unfortunately, eye movement recordings have demonstrated that abnormal eye movements are secondary to word identification and comprehension problems, and not the converse.

Eyes do not track when a person reads. Instead, the eyes make short rapid eye movements called saccades. Saccades vary in length with intermittent fixations of various times. When one reads from left to right, most saccades are oriented to the right with some saccades showing reversal of direction, equating to a reader going backwards to reread something they could not decipher or did not understand. Readers with dyslexia have abnormal saccades on eye movement recordings and fixation patterns similar to the beginning reader but show normal saccadic eye movements when the content is adjusted for ability.[10,11] The abnormal saccades in readers with dyslexia appear to be the result, not the cause, of their reading disability.[10–13]

LEARNING DISABILITIES

The following is an excerpt of a joint statement from the American Academy of Pediatrics (Section on Ophthalmology, Council on Children with Disabilities), the American Academy of Ophthalmology, the American Association for Pediatric Ophthalmology and Strabismus, and the American Association of Certified Orthoptists regarding learning disabilities, dyslexia, and vision therapy. The entire policy statement has an in-depth well-referenced explanation of the role the visual system plays in reading.[14] The excerpt reads as follows:

Dyslexia

Approximately 80% of people with learning disabilities have dyslexia. The terms "reading disability" and "dyslexia" are often used interchangeably in the literature. Dyslexia is a primary reading disorder and results from a written word processing abnormality in the brain.[1] It is characterized by difficulties with accurate and/or fluent sight word recognition and by poor spelling and decoding abilities. These difficulties are unexpected in relation to the child's other cognitive skills. Dyslexia has been identified as having a strong genetic basis. Recent genetic-linkage studies have identified many loci at which dyslexia-related genes are encoded.

Approximately 40% of siblings, children, or parents of an affected individual will have dyslexia.

Dyslexia is identified in some people early in their lives but in others is not diagnosed until much later, when more complex reading and writing skills are required. People with dyslexia can be very bright and may be gifted in math, science, the arts, or even in unexpected areas such as writing. Dyslexia should be separated from other secondary forms of reading difficulties caused by visual or hearing disorders, mental retardation, and experiential or instructional deficits. Early reading difficulties may be caused by experiential and instructional deficits. It is important to identify and address such causes of secondary reading difficulties.

...English is a phonemically complex language in which the 26 letters of the alphabet create 44 sounds, or phonemes, in approximately 70 letter combinations. The phonemic complexity of an alphabet-based language corresponds to the prevalence of dyslexia, pointing to the linguistic origin of dyslexia. Reading involves the integration of multiple factors related to a person's experience, ability, and neurologic functioning. Most people with dyslexia have a neurobiological deficit in the processing of the sound structure of language, called a phonemic deficit, which exists despite relatively intact overall language abilities. Children with more severe forms of dyslexia may have a second deficit in naming letters, numbers, and pictures, creating a double deficit, or they may have problems with their attention or working memory. Other children may have trouble orienting, recognizing, and remembering letter combinations. This difficulty may be a neuromaturational delay that improves with development. Importantly, the definition of dyslexia does not include reversal of letters or words or mirror reading or writing, which are commonly held misconceptions.

Controversies

Because they are difficult for the public to understand and for educators to treat, learning disabilities have spawned a wide variety of controversial and scientifically unsupported alternative treatments, including vision therapy. Scientific evidence of effectiveness should be the basis for treatment accommodations. Treatments that have inadequate scientific proof of efficacy should be discouraged. Ineffective, controversial methods of treatment such as vision therapy may give parents and teachers a false sense of security that a child's learning difficulties are being addressed, may waste family and/or school resources, and may delay proper instruction or remediation.

Currently, there is inadequate scientific evidence to support the view that subtle eye or visual problems, including abnormal focusing, jerky eye movements, misaligned or crossed eyes, binocular dysfunction, visual-motor dysfunction, visual perceptual difficulties, or hypothetical difficulties with laterality or "trouble crossing the midline" of the visual field, cause learning disabilities. Statistically, children with dyslexia or related learning disabilities have the same visual function and ocular health as children without such conditions. Because visual problems do not underlie dyslexia, approaches designed to improve visual function by training are misdirected. Other than convergence-insufficiency treatment, scientific evidence does not support the assumption that vision therapy is capable of correcting subtle visual defects, nor does it prove eye exercises or behavioral vision therapy to be effective direct or indirect treatments for learning disabilities. Detailed review of the literature supporting vision therapy reveals that most of the information is poorly validated, because it relies on anecdotes, poorly designed studies, and poorly controlled or uncontrolled studies. Their reported benefits can often be explained by the placebo effect or by the traditional educational remedial techniques with which they are usually combined. There is currently no evidence that children who participate in vision therapy are more responsive to educational instruction than are children who do not participate. Thus, current evidence is of poor scientific quality and does not provide adequate scientific evidence that vision training is a necessary primary or adjunctive therapy.

The pediatrician is the valued advisor of parents, and often parents seek the advice of their pediatrician regarding visual therapy. Unfortunately, the children considering vision therapy often face many hurdles including learning disabilities with or without behavioral and physical disabilities. The author has observed that very dedicated parents are searching for therapies and interventions that can help their children. They are easy "targets" for unproven therapies that promise to help their children. The author's approach is to educate parents about the lack of scientific data for vision therapy for the treatment of learning disabilities and perform a complete eye examination to make sure there is not any ocular pathologic abnormality that could be limiting vision or creating additional problems (eg, diplopia or CI) that might hinder educational interventions for learning disabilities. Once the author is certain that the patient has normal ocular health and she has educated the parents, the author gives them her blessing to pursue any vision therapy that they want to try. There are anecdotal stories of improvement. The cost is out-of-pocket and usually the parents' hopes are not realized.

Completely contrary to the joint excerpt from the American Academy of Pediatrics, the American Academy of Ophthalmology, the American Association for Pediatric Ophthalmology and Strabismus, and the American Association of Certified Orthoptists, the American Optometric Association[15] asserts in their policy statement, "Learning to read and reading for information require efficient visual abilities. The eyes must team precisely, focus clearly, and track quickly and accurately across the page. These processes must be coordinated with the perceptual and memory aspects of vision, which in turn must combine with linguistic processing for comprehension. To provide reliable information, this must occur with precise timing. Inefficient or poorly developed vision requires individuals to divide their attention between the task and the involved visual abilities." Decoding and comprehension failure, rather than a primary abnormality of the oculomotor control systems, are responsible for slow reading, increased duration of fixations, and increased backward saccades.[16] Finally, children with saccadic disorders do not show an increased likelihood of dyslexia.[17] As indicated above, dyslexia is not correlated with eye or eye movement abnormalities.[18–21]

SUMMARY

Convergence therapy is a scientifically proven treatment for CI. There is currently a PEDIG (Pediatric Eye Disease Investigator Group) study underway to assess the various forms of therapy (CITS). They are recruiting patients and this study will give additional information about the success of various forms of convergence therapy. Vision therapy for problems other than CI is unproven, and ophthalmologists and most optometrists adhere to the scientific principle that abnormal saccades are the result of learning disabilities that affect reading, and not the cause. Therefore, there is no role for vision therapy in children with learning disabilities or cognitive disabilities.

REFERENCES

1. Scheiman M, Mitchell GL, Cotter S, et al, The Convergence Insufficiency Treatment Trial (CITT) Study Group. A randomized clinical trial of treatments for convergence insufficiency in children. Arch Ophthalmol 2005;123:14–24.
2. Rouse MW, Borsting E, Hyman L, et al. Frequency of convergence insufficiency among fifth and sixth graders. Optom Vis Sci 1999;76(9):643–9.
3. Letourneau JE, Ducic S. Prevalence of convergence insufficiency among elementary school children. Can J Optom 1988;50:194–7.
4. Borsting EJ, Rouse MW, Mitchell GL, et al. Validity and reliability of the revised convergence insufficiency symptom survey in children aged 9-18 years. Optom Vis Sci 2003;80:832–8.
5. Mitchell G, Scheiman M, Borsting E, et al. Evaluation of a symptom survey for convergence insufficiency patients. Optom Vis Sci 2001;12:37.
6. Borsting E, Rouse MW, DeLand PN. Prospective comparison of convergence insufficiency and normal binocular children on CIRS symptom surveys. Convergence Insufficiency and Reading Study (CIRS) Group. Optom Vis Sci 1999;76(4):221–8.
7. Borsting E, Rouse MW, DeLand PN, et al. Association of symptoms and convergence and accommodative insufficiency in school-age children. Optometry 2003;74:25–34.
8. Serna A, Rogers DL, McGregor ML, et al. Treatment of symptomatic convergence insufficiency with a home-based computer orthoptic exercise program. J AAPOS 2011;15:140–3.
9. Cacho Martínez P, García Muñoz A, Ruiz-Cantero MT. Treatment of accommodative and nonstrabismic binocular dysfunctions: a systematic review. Optometry 2009;80(12):702–16.
10. Metzger RL, Werner DB. Use of visual training for reading disabilities: a review. Pediatrics 1984;73(6):824–9.
11. Levine MD. Reading disability: do the eyes have it? Pediatrics 1984;73(6):869–70.
12. Solan HA. An appraisal of the Irlen technique of correcting reading disorders using tinted overlays and tinted lenses. J Learn Disabil 1990;23(10):621–6.
13. Evans BJ, Drasdo N. Tinted lenses and related therapies for learning disabilities–a review. Ophthalmic Physiol Opt 1991;11(3):206–17.
14. Joint statement: learning disabilities, dyslexia, and vision–reaffirmed 2014 AAP, AAPOS, AACO and AAO Hoskins Center for quality eye care. 2014. Available at: http://one.aao.org/clinical-statement/joint-statement-learning-disabilities-dyslexia-vis. Accessed February 9, 2014.
15. American Optometric Association. Position statement on vision therapy. J Am Optom Assoc 1985;56:782–3. Available at: http://www.aoa.org/optometrists/education-and-training/clinical-care/vision-therapy. Accessed February 9, 2014.
16. Hoyt CS. Visual training and reading. Am Orthopt J 1999;49:23–5.
17. Hodgetts DJ, Simon JW, Sibila TA, et al. Normal reading despite limited eye movements. J AAPOS 1998;2(3):182–3.
18. Vellutino FR, Fletcher JM, Snowling MJ, et al. Specific reading disability (dyslexia): what have we learned in the past four decades? J Child Psychol Psychiatry 2004;45(1):2–40.
19. Olitsky SE, Nelson LB. Reading disorders in children. Pediatr Clin North Am 2003;50(1):213–24.
20. Beauchamp GR, Kosmorsky G. Learning disabilities: update comment on the visual system. Pediatr Clin North Am 1987;34(6):1439–46.

21. American Academy of Ophthalmology Complementary Therapy Task Force. Complementary therapy assessment: vision therapy for learning disabilities. San Francisco (CA): American Academy of Ophthalmology; 2001. Available at: http://one.aao.org/CE/PracticeGuidelines/Therapy.aspx. Accessed September 26, 2006.

Index

Note: Page numbers of article titles are in **boldface** type.

Printed and bound by CPI Group (UK) Ltd, Croydon, CR0 4YY

08/06/2025

01896875-0008